Despair Today – Hope for Tomorrow

A mother's story of resilience on the journey of advocacy for her son with disability and mental illness

Elizabeth Patterson

First published by Busybird Publishing 2025

Copyright © 2025 Elizabeth Patterson

ISBN
Print: 978-1-923501-16-4

This work is copyright. Apart from any use permitted under the *Copyright Act 1968*, no part of this publication may be reproduced, stored in a retrieval system or transmitted in any form or by any means, electronic, mechanical, photocopying, recording or otherwise, without the prior written permission of Elizabeth Patterson.

The information in this book is based on the author's experiences and opinions. The author and publisher disclaim responsibility for any adverse consequences that may result from use of the information contained herein. Permission to use any external content has been sought by the author. Any breaches will be rectified in further editions of the book.

Cover Image: Alan Swann
Cover design: Busybird Publishing
Layout and typesetting: Busybird Publishing

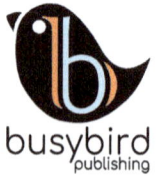

Busybird Publishing
2/118 Para Road
Montmorency, Victoria
Australia 3094
www.busybird.com.au

Contents

Preface i

New Beginnings
Journeying into the unknown 1

Cradles and Chaos
Navigating the storms of new life and mental turmoil 5

Rewriting Tomorrow
Embracing family, faith and community in response to a devastating diagnosis 10

Leaving the Nest
Learning to fly and thrive again 17

Confronting the Boundaries
Negotiating the continuum of inclusive education 25

Unforeseen Blessings
The gift of allies on our path 31

Passport to Possibilities
Experiencing the joys and jitters of traveling 39

Holding Together
Enduring the burden of deficiencies in mental health services 47

Photos 54

At the Crossroads
Bearing the burden of caregiver decisions 67

Negotiating the NDIS
Traversing the everchanging landscape 72

The Woof Whisperers
Encountering the power of canine companionship 80

On the Brink
Balancing on a knife edge of physical and mental health relapse 87

Taking a Stance
Advocating amidst the shadows of recrimination 93

Fragile Moments
Creating calm amidst the tempest 102

Knocking on Empty
Refilling the resilience tank 109

Divine Assurance
Finding strength through adversity 115

Preface

This is my story of life with James, my son who has severe disabilities and mental illness. I tell it primarily from the perspective of his mother, while also incorporating my experiences as a nurse and academic. Rather than following a chronological format, this narrative consists of a series of vignettes that depict significant life events and experiences.

For over forty years, I have experienced a wide spectrum of emotions, ranging from overwhelming love, joy, compassion, tolerance, and patience to anxiety, fear, dread, despair, and sadness. These moments have fostered courage and resilience — qualities often unrecognised in the moment but later illuminated by the realisation that I can do this, again and again, if I have to for James' sake. As a Christian, I also reflect on the struggles and frustrations I have had with God regarding suffering, as well as on my faith and the profound hope I hold for James beyond his earthly life.

Life can be a blend of richness and bleakness, and sometimes it has only taken a shared moment or an understanding nod from another person to restore a sense of balance to my perspective. A wise pastor once advised that in moments of darkness, we should pause, reflect, and consider before reacting. This is often difficult to do in the moment, but it becomes easier with practice. Additionally, finding a bit of humor in the situation has been beneficial for my soul!

James was born in May 1981 in King George V Memorial Hospital in Sydney. Within 24 hours, my fear that 'something was not right' was confirmed when a young doctor approached my bed the morning after his birth and told me that staff had observed James having a seizure during the night, and that he was 'floppy' and unable to suck.

He had been placed in the Neonatal Intensive Care Unit (NICU) and there began a battery of tests to determine the cause. Six weeks later, James was discharged from the NICU still floppy, hard to feed and with no definitive diagnosis, just 'perhaps it's atypical cerebral palsy.'

During the first two years of James' life, it became increasingly apparent that my husband was mentally unstable, which often put James and me in danger from his unpredictable violent behaviour. Under very difficult circumstances, James and I left him in Sydney and moved interstate.

A consultation with a neurologist at the Cerebral Palsy League in Brisbane finally revealed a diagnosis for James, Prader-Willi Syndrome (PWS):

> 'A genetic multisystem disorder characterised during infancy by lethargy, diminished muscle tone (hypotonia), a weak suck and feeding difficulties with poor weight gain and growth and other hormone deficiency. In childhood, features of this disorder include short stature, small genitals and an excessive appetite. Affected individuals do not feel satisfied after completing a meal (satiety). Without intervention, overeating can lead to onset of life-threatening obesity. The food compulsion requires constant supervision... All individuals with PWS have some cognitive impairment that ranges from low normal intelligence with learning disabilities to mild to moderate intellectual disability. Behavioral problems are common and can include temper tantrums, obsessive/compulsive behavior and skin picking. Motor milestones and language development are often delayed.' (National Organization for Rare Disorders website).

Fortunately for us, there was an Early Intervention Teaching Program in Tweed Heads, close to where we were living, which provided excellent support for James' physical, cognitive and social development and facilitated his attendance at a local pre-school. James attended mainstream primary schools with assistance from special education teachers, but his enrolment in mainstream secondary education was cut short in his first year because of the inability of teachers to manage the challenging behaviours associated with PWS. He was then transferred to a school for children with intellectual and other disabilities.

On leaving this school, James gained supported employment in the laundry of one of the Sheraton hotels but, by age 21, he was exhibiting signs and symptoms of psychosis and endured his first admission to an acute psychiatric ward – to be followed by numerous other admissions over the course of his life, which ended his ability to be employed. Subsequent to unemployment, James has attended a centre-based day program and benefitted from other community access support services for people with disabilities.

Just prior to James turning 30, we moved to Melbourne from the Gold Coast. After several admissions to acute psychiatric wards and with very little government support to help me manage his care, at 33, James moved into Specialist Disability Accommodation run by the Victorian Department of Health and Human Services, later to be managed by another provider under the National Disability Insurance Scheme.

Each of these life stages and changes has brought struggles and triumphs and, along the way, I have learnt what it means to be an advocate for a vulnerable and often disempowered person; rewarding if it results in an improved quality of life for James but, at other times, oh so costly to my own wellbeing.

I have written this book because I wanted to document the journey partly for my own healing but also to inspire others to keep going, not give up, trust their instincts, call out injustice when they experience it, lean on others when needed and acknowledge the inner strength they have. Although the journey has been painful, I have been blessed with discovering Christian faith, having a loving and supportive family and faith community, friends I may never have made on a different life journey and compassionate and committed disability support workers who have partnered with me to enhance James' quality of life whenever possible.

New Beginnings

Journeying into the unknown

It is early in 1981 and I am in the last months of pregnancy with my first child. I am lying back on the couch one evening watching the television and a new documentary series begins, *A Matter of Chance*. It is presented by Anne Deveson and produced by ABC-TV as a contribution to the International Year of the Disabled which had been proclaimed by the United Nations that year. The series is introduced as 'looking at the problems and aspirations of the disabled in Australia – the people most of us prefer to ignore.'

Oh dear, do I want to watch this?

> *Before I formed you in the womb I knew you,*
> *before you were born I set you apart.*
> **Jeremiah 1:5**

Surprisingly, 44 years on I still have such vivid memories of that experience even though I did not know at the time that I was carrying a child who would have multiple special needs. Any prospective parent would probably have some misgivings about watching a documentary on disabilities, but I felt particularly troubled as I was already feeling apprehensive about bringing a baby into a marriage that was rocky to say the least.

My husband, Gordon, had been mentally unravelling over the past year. He had resigned from working as a secondary school maths teacher, and had started working in a bakery in the early hours of the morning so that he could spend the rest of the day producing oil paintings that he envisaged would bring him fame and fortune. He was financing this by selling off our possessions – first the car, and then items of furniture. He had also converted part of the house into a studio in which he had birds flying around. Friends had stopped visiting because of his ever-increasing bizarre behaviours and his family appeared to have their heads firmly buried in the sand.

I was feeling very alone and vulnerable.

Adding to my consternation were comments from my sister, who was a midwife, that the baby's faint, almost indiscernible movements in utero were concerning. Although I was a registered nurse, I had not done midwifery so knowledge of 'normal pregnancy' was framed within the experiences of mothers I knew. Routine ultrasounds had not revealed any abnormalities.

But I was left with a feeling of disquiet.

The baby was due in late April, and as a week and then another week passed with no signs of an imminent birth, my anxiety increased until the early hours of 13th May when labour began and I presented to the King George V Memorial Hospital, accompanied by Gordon. The first assessment by the admitting midwife revealed foetal distress and resulted in an immediate phone call to the obstetrician who instructed her to commence medication to speed up the process to get the baby out. Some hours later, the obstetrician appeared and after a quick examination said he would return to perform a forceps delivery.

Initial excitement and an expectation of a natural birth quickly turned to growing panic.

At 3:50pm James was born, snowy haired and perfectly formed, yet quiet and motionless – no cries, no kicking or squirming, just flaccid. Despite reassurances of 'he will be okay', James was taken away to the Special Care Nursery for observation and I was allowed one visit later that evening. He looked angelic and peaceful so I went to sleep hopeful that, by the next morning, everything would be alright – but still felt a sense of foreboding in the pit of my stomach.

Early the next morning, I was awakened by a young doctor who told me that nursing staff had observed James having a seizure and that they were very concerned because he was still very floppy, couldn't suck and had not cried at all. They had commenced tube feeds and transferred him to the Neonatal Intensive Care Unit (NICU).

This can't be happening!

My memories of the next six weeks include daily visits to James in the NICU, sometimes lasting all day and with endless tests and assessments by a variety of specialists. There were also visits from relatives and friends bearing gifts and platitudes of 'everything will be fine.'

Gordon was in a persistent downward spiral of habitual marijuana smoking and incoherent ramblings from the I Ching and other sources of eastern mysticism. I was anxious going into the hospital not knowing what I would be confronted with, frightened of approaching doctors because of what they might declare and terrified of going home each night because that might be the night Gordon 'lost it' completely.

Day after day, I waited and hoped for an explanation of what was causing James' hypotonia (floppiness) and lack of responsiveness because, in knowing, I thought I could do something to fix it. I faithfully engaged in all the exercises and strategies shown to me by the physiotherapists to try and stimulate enough muscle tone in James to enable him to suck from a bottle of breast milk that I expressed every day.

Finally came the day – after six weeks – when he could suck enough to consume his daily requirements (even though each feed took about an hour) and he was discharged home. None of the tests – brain CT, EEG, blood and urine pathology – identified any abnormalities, so there was no diagnosis and therefore no prognosis. The only explanation provided was that he could have a form of cerebral palsy, but his presentation was not characteristic of that.

The journey to hospital on 13th May had started with excitement and an expectation of new beginnings as a family which, hopefully, might have restored Gordon's mental stability – but it was not to be. Instead, six weeks later I took a baby home from the NICU who required much more care than anticipated, an unknown reason for his condition and a husband who was mentally escalating out of control.

The unease I had experienced earlier in the year while watching *A Matter of Chance* was becoming a reality.

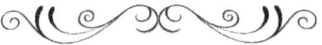

Cradles and Chaos

Navigating the storms of new life and mental turmoil

It is Mother's Day 1983. James and I are sitting on a plane on the tarmac in Sydney waiting for take-off to Melbourne. I had purchased return tickets, but I knew we would not be returning. With a churning stomach and rapidly beating heart, I had convinced Gordon that I needed to introduce James to his Aunty Sue, Uncle Norm and three cousins Nick, Daniel and Stephen and that we would be back in a few days. Without announcement, two uniformed officers from the Australian Federal Police boarded the plane and stopped next to my seat. They said there was a very agitated man in the departure lounge wanting to talk to me. My response was quick and firm, 'no, I am scared he will abscond with my son.'

Many are the plans in a person's heart,
but it is the Lord's purpose that prevails.
Proverbs 19:21

For James' wellbeing, our safety, and to find refuge with my family interstate, we had to leave Sydney.

Since James' discharge from hospital nearly two years previously, my life had become a mixture of attending to his special needs and navigating my way round Gordon's fluctuating moods, demands and controlling behaviour.

In the first few months after James' discharge from the NICU, I had to set the alarm every three hours, day and night, to feed him because he didn't cry or display any signs of hunger – he just slept peacefully or gazed quietly and intently around his surroundings. On referral from the hospital, I had started taking James to the Spastic Centre (later to be called the Cerebral Palsy League) on the North Shore of Sydney – a fair distance from where we lived in Balmain – to start physiotherapy, so a regime of exercises and stimulating activities was added to the daily routine. James gradually became more responsive to his environment and feeding times started to improve.

During this time, Gordon continued working at the local bakery – leaving home at 3am and returning at 7am. Some days he would arrive home calm and eager to engage with James, and at other times I knew it was going to be a difficult day as soon as he walked in. He would be agitated and argumentative, often accusing the obstetrician of harming James or asserting that he could cure whatever was wrong with him by consulting the I Ching – all while under the influence of marijuana.

Although I had attended Sunday school as a child and gone through the process of Confirmation as a teenager, I had no real concept of what it meant to be a Christian. I had Bible knowledge, but no heart affiliation. Despite this, something in my inner being felt very uncomfortable with all of this I Ching activity.

Not unexpectedly, Gordon was fired from the bakery. He didn't reveal why and he didn't seem bothered by it, nor did he express any desire to find alternative employment or take any responsibility for seeking financial support. Consequently, I returned to work as a registered nurse, only doing evening shifts from 1:00-10:00pm so that I could continue taking James to his therapy sessions in the mornings. I had no doubt that Gordon loved James and would try his best to look after him in my absence, but it still filled me with apprehension that he would become consumed by his obsessive need to paint and forget to feed him or, worse than that, become agitated and leave James alone in the house while he went in search of a supply of 'dope'.

When James was three months old, I noticed what appeared to be an inguinal hernia, which was confirmed by the GP and a paediatric surgeon. He was booked for surgery at the Royal Children's Hospital in Camperdown, and my lasting memory of that day was waiting and hoping that he would cry because that would reassure me that his brain was more responsive to stimuli than he had previously demonstrated.

He did!

My obvious excitement must have seemed very odd to the other parents waiting in the recovery area for their child to return from surgery. No doubt some would have thought, 'what an uncaring mother.'

The next big hiccup eventuated when a therapist at the Spastic Centre suggested that James may be hearing impaired, in addition to his other developmental delays, because he didn't instantly startle at unexpected noises close to him and he wasn't 'babbling' as expected for his age – he was 10 months old. Off we went to another assessment, this time at the National Acoustics Laboratory, where it was verified that he had mild to moderate hearing loss in both ears. Soon after, he was fitted with hearing aids.

Although this was another blow, it had a silver lining because we were introduced to a wonderful lady called Joan from the Shepherd Centre – an organisation established by the Shepherd family who had two profoundly hearing-impaired children. The aim of this organisation was to empower babies and toddlers with hearing loss to develop spoken language, as well as listening and social skills, through a home visiting early intervention program.

Joan was an absolute delight and positive influence in our lives. I looked forward to her weekly visits and to the outings we went on to expose James to the natural sounds of the environment, animal noises at the zoo and the spoken words of other toddlers and adults. The outings included other families with hearing impaired children so they provided mutual support, understanding and social engagement – things that I would otherwise have missed out on because my family were all interstate and old friends were fast disappearing from our lives.

This was but one of the many 'cradles' I later came to recognise as God's way of redeeming our story. That is, his provision of supports and safe spaces to transform our difficult situation to a more hopeful one.

It is interesting to think back to events that had a really heartbreaking impact and to be able now to reflect on them with a different perspective. One such event was when a longtime friend of Gordon's, on seeing James wearing hearing aids for the first time, exclaimed 'he looks like he's got two bananas stuck to his head!'

At the time, tears of hurt and anger were just held back, but now I can envisage his reaction as that of someone who was uncomfortable and ill-equipped when confronted with 'difference' and so used humour as a coping mechanism. It still happens 43 years on from that event – but, thankfully, not as often.

After a particularly frightening experience when Gordon literally dragged James and me from our beds on a cold wet night because he wanted to find a circus somewhere (there were none in Sydney at the time), I decided enough was enough – James and I had to get away from this ongoing, unreasonable and dangerous situation. I knew that my parents, who lived in northern NSW, were visiting my sister Sue and her family in Melbourne for a few weeks so I took the opportunity to flee with James to a safe haven and family support.

Fortunately, the Australian Federal Police who had confronted me on the plane in Sydney were sufficiently convinced of our dire situation to let us continue with our escape.

Rewriting Tomorrow

Embracing family, faith and community in response to a devastating diagnosis

It is an afternoon in July 1983. Mum, James and I are driving from Brisbane back to the Tweed Coast after spending the morning in medical consultations at the Cerebral Palsy League. It is deathly quiet, no radio playing and no conversation – if I were to utter a word the floodgates would open. Mum looks stricken and James is sleeping in his car seat. The words 'it's Prader-Willi Syndrome' keep repeating in my mind.

The disturbing textbook words and images of grossly obese children keep playing on a never-ending spool.

Just concentrate on the road.

> *God is our shelter and our strength,*
> *always ready to help in times of trouble.*
> **Psalm 46:1**

Two months previously, James and I had arrived in Melbourne after fleeing from Sydney with a small overnight bag and about $50 in hand. It was a challenging few weeks with mixed emotions and decisions to be made about where we would make our new home: with my sister and her family in Melbourne, or with my mother and father in northern NSW at Terranora. After many unnerving phone calls from Gordon, I decided that I could not subject my sister and her young children to the possibility of ongoing harassment from him so decided we would return with Mum and Dad to Terranora. Another important factor in making this decision was knowing that there was an early intervention teaching program (EITP) in Tweed Heads, just a short drive from Terranora.

After a long drive from Melbourne to Terranora (via Canberra to visit old friends) we arrived in the afternoon to find Gordon emerging from the rockery in the front garden! He informed us that he had hitch-hiked up from Sydney a few days earlier and was staying in a motel in Tweed Heads awaiting our arrival. Dad ushered Mum, James and me inside the house and then drove Gordon to the motel, saying we would discuss the situation with him the next day. That event was the start of a six-year period of visitations from Gordon – some unexpected, and some sanctioned by the family court – all resulting in anxiety and fear over what the next visit would entail.

James was soon enrolled in the EITP where we met our next gem – Judith, the teacher. Three times a week, he spent two hours with Judith and three other children having wonderful fun while learning to socialise, communicate and develop his fine and gross motor skills. Having the EITP situated in the community health centre enabled access to – and support from – allied health therapists and psychologists during or after the early intervention teaching sessions. It was during a session with the physiotherapist that she suggested we should make an appointment with the Cerebral Palsy Centre in Brisbane to be reviewed by a neurologist.

That appointment started with an examination by a neurology registrar who gave my mother and I great hope when he said that it was highly unlikely that James had cerebral palsy and that with continued physiotherapy, his muscle tone would improve and he would probably then develop normally. He assured us that James did not appear to have any cognitive impairment and as long as he wore his hearing aids and engaged in speech therapy, he would also be able to communicate well.

What a relief – but it didn't last long!

One hour later, the next examination was conducted by the consultant neurologist who took one look at James and then asked, 'how much does he like and demand food?' James, after initially being hard to feed and slow to gain weight, was now quite chubby. I responded very excitedly, 'oh, he loves his food; can't get enough of it – he rolls across the floor to his highchair and rattles it all the time!'

'Mmmmm, thought so,' said the neurologist, 'I'm pretty sure I know what he has, but will have to confirm with a chromosome test. I think it's Prader-Willi Syndrome.'

As he was saying this, he had pulled a textbook off the shelf titled *Congenital Syndromes,* placed it on the desk in front of us and opened it to the relevant pages headed 'Prader-Willi Syndrome (PWS)'. As I quickly read through it, some of the words seemed to fly off the page at me:

- no cure
- intellectually disabled
- insatiable appetite
- morbid obesity
- challenging behaviours
- infertile
- shortened lifespan.

The description of the syndrome was accompanied by photos of affected children and adults – cute little babies looking just like James, then obese children to grossly obese, short adults. The photos reminded me of the dreadful images that used to promote circus freak shows in a previous century.

Flummoxed by the contradictory prognoses given that morning and too shocked to ask many questions, we left hurriedly with the name of a family living in Brisbane from whom we could seek advice, as they had a daughter with PWS. After receiving therapy services from the Cerebral Palsy Centre in Sydney, James' new diagnosis meant there would be no further support from the Brisbane centre.

The next day after relaying the experience and diagnosis to Judith, she paused for a moment and then said, 'James is the same little boy today as he was yesterday; we now know what we are dealing with so let's find out all we can about PWS, make a plan to help him and get on with it.'

This has been a mantra that has stuck with me.

Part of that plan included a consultation with a dietitian and there began a lifetime for James of monitoring, limiting, evaluating and obsessing about every mouthful of food and drink he ingested. In turn, this also instigated changes for all family members around James when food was involved – regular meals and snacks, birthdays, Christmas, eating out and just about all social events.

PWS necessitates a state of food security for all involved!

While this is constant and stressful, it has also provided for some very creative and humorous family events. One of these involved my sister Sue, her three small children, James and me. We had all been for a ride on a miniature train and, on alighting, saw a mobile doughnut van. Needless to say, Sue's children all wanted a doughnut – which resulted in each of us taking turns to sneak behind the van and scoff a doughnut while another shielded James from the sight and kept him occupied.

I still have visions of jam being hurriedly wiped from chins.

Another event that caused a great deal of mirth arose during a farm stay holiday that James had been on with a family support group respite service. He asked the farmer to show him the cows that produced skim milk and couldn't understand why everyone was laughing so much. Since his diagnosis, we had been quite open with James about what foods were suitable for him and he knew that he was allowed reduced fat dairy products and he knew that milk came from cows so he figured there must be 'skim milk cows'.

Smart kid!

Judith's compassionate and pragmatic support of James over the four years that he was associated with the EITP enabled him to develop to the best of his capacity and be successfully integrated into a local pre-school. By the time he started he was talking, walking, playing appropriately with his peers and able to recognise and name numbers, letters and short words.

At the same time, I had joined the North Coast Family Support Group, comprising of family members of children with disabilities, and enjoyed their support and encouragement while contributing to fundraising activities to finance the rapidly growing EITP.

Living with my parents not only provided me with help to manage James and all his therapies, but also gave me the opportunity to return to part-time work as a registered nurse at Tweed Heads Private Hospital. While I was working there, the Director of Nursing encouraged me to enroll in postgraduate distance education at the University of New England. I had completed a Bachelor of Science before commencing nursing studies, so I was able to enter a Graduate Diploma in Nursing Education without having to undertake a bridging course. Studying again gave me a renewed interest and purpose in life, apart from being the mother of a child with special needs.

Living on the beautiful north coast of NSW with close proximity to beaches, waterways and the hinterland provided a wonderful environment and attraction for interstate friends and family to holiday with us which greatly enriched our lives. James thrived with the attention he got from his Nanna and Pa and with the companionship of two of his cousins, Lee and Tim, who were of similar age and lived close by on the Gold Coast with their Mum, Cherry – my younger sister.

James' early years at primary school were spent initially at Terranora and then at Banora Point when we downsized from a house on acreage to a smaller property nearby. James loved both schools and, although developmentally delayed, he kept up with his peers in a mainstream setting and with no additional teacher aide assistance. This was due to the patient, caring and dedicated teachers he had but also, in no small part, to the hours of informal and experiential teaching he received from his Nanna and Pa who were devoted to him.

James would get into bed with his Nanna every morning for reading – sometimes it would be children's Bible stories, and other times it would be practising letters, words and numbers. His Pa took him for walks along the Tweed River at Tumbulgum so they could watch the car ferry cross the river and then feed the ferry master's pet cockatoo thistles that they had collected along the way. Pa used every opportunity to teach James the names of trees and plants they saw, as well as listening out for different bird sounds. James also got his love of watching sport from his Pa – they would watch the AFL and cricket together, with Pa teaching James the rules of the games.

I had experienced periods of numbing fear and desolation going through the trauma of James' birth, separation from Gordon and then James' diagnosis and, although feeling supported by a loving family, teachers, therapists and new friends, I was also aware of an inner void; something I could not quite work out how to fill. I partially addressed this emptiness by immersing myself in easing the suffering of others through nursing, and satisfying my hunger for learning through studying.

Nevertheless, I had a sense there was something still missing.

I had become aware that my mother and older sister Sue in Melbourne had started attending church, and both were engaged in Bible study groups. At the time I thought, 'that's nice, each to their own… a bit like joining a book club or something.'

I also remember thinking, 'I hope they don't start preaching at me!'

Yet, at the same time, I felt comforted hearing that they and their Christian friends were praying for us.

One day, I decided to go with Mum to her Bible study group called Know Your Bible (KYB). It comprised a group of ladies, all older than me but instantly I felt accepted by these wise, nurturing, and loving women. Over time, with study, discussion and reflection came a slow dawning of who Jesus was and what he had done for me.

I came to accept that he was not just the historical figure who had healed the sick and befriended the marginalised but, more importantly, he had subjected himself to an agonising death to reconcile me to my creator, God. I experienced a profound astonishment that I had never understood this before. From that revelation, I developed a hunger to learn more about the Christian faith, which I satisfied by undertaking the Bethel Bible Series and then much later another Bible study under the auspices of Bible Study Fellowship.

From then on, Christianity has given me a foundation on which to build a framework of support, resilience and hope, even through times of despair and perceived helplessness. I have recognised that God's enabling power is at work in my life, long before I am aware of it, and that his providence has brought me into mutually blessed relationships.

I believe that this enabling power has often been initiated by others' faith and intercessory prayer, particularly when profound suffering has caused me to question my own faith.

Over a period of six years – from fleeing Sydney to making a new home in northern NSW, confronting a lifelong devastating condition, enduring traumatic family court decisions, and getting on with the ordinary business of an extraordinary life – James and I settled into our tribes.

Leaving the Nest

Learning to fly and thrive again

It is late morning on 6 December 1989 and I am working at Tweed Heads Private Hospital in the High Dependency Unit. The phone rings and it is Mum. She says 'Elizabeth, I think you need to come home. Bill (Gordon's father) has just phoned to say Gordon has died. He jumped off the Sydney Harbour Bridge.'

My head spins, thoughts race and feelings fluctuate. I have a sense of overwhelming relief mixed with sadness for his family and grief for a life so talented but tortured.

But those who trust in the Lord for help will find their strength renewed.
They will rise on wings like eagles;
they will run and not grow weary;
they will walk and not grow weak.
Isaiah 40:31

What had led to this horrendous event?

After James and I relocated to Terranora to live with Mum and Dad, Gordon had initially randomly appeared at our front door every few months after booking himself into a motel in Tweed Heads. Dad took it upon himself to supervise Gordon's time with James, usually spent on the foreshore of the Tweed Heads boat harbour. Gordon always arrived with hand-carved wooden toys that he had made for James.

I had heard from Gordon's parents that he had been hospitalised a few times as an involuntary patient in a psychiatric ward after public disturbances and altercations with police. It soon became obvious to us when Gordon visited whether he was on medication or not – medicated he was over-weight and calm, not medicated he was under-weight and agitated.

Medicated Gordon resulted in a relaxed time spent with James, but unmedicated Gordon was a nightmare experience – loud incoherent ramblings, wild eyed confrontations with bystanders and occasions when I would find him lying under my car outside the hospital where I worked, so I couldn't drive away.

The last of the nightmare experiences involved Gordon trying to run off with James after punching my father. Fortunately, other people in the park witnessed the event, gave chase and phoned the police, who intervened.

After that episode, I sought legal advice as to what to do to protect James and the rest of the family. This resulted in several family court hearings, most of which Gordon attended. One such hearing is seared into my memory. Gordon stood before the magistrate and recited an A. A. Milne poem over and over to every question put to him, saying 'Christopher Robin goes hoppity, hoppity, hoppity hop…'

The magistrate acknowledged that Gordon was mentally unwell and advised him to get a barrister to represent him at future hearings. To say I was gobsmacked is an understatement! While understanding the Family Court's desire to afford children the opportunity to routinely engage with both parents, I was perplexed by the apparent indifference to Gordon's unstable and often unsafe behaviour.

After representations by Gordon's barrister, the magistrate ordered that continuing access visits to James be allowed, but were to be supervised by a psychologist known to James. This arrangement continued for several monthly visits until the psychologist reported back to the Family Court that it was not safe for James or himself to continue.

After being told that he could not have access to James until a psychiatrist deemed him to be mentally stable, Gordon voluntarily accepted further inpatient psychiatric care. During the last of these inpatient stays, Gordon phoned me and appeared to have insight into his condition and the lifelong impact this would have on him. I recall him saying 'I'm not good… I'm going mad… I can't think properly on these tablets… I can't write music anymore or paint.'

It was not long after this conversation and discharge from this hospital stay that he ended his life.

During the last six years of his life, Gordon had taught himself to read music and play classical guitar. He transformed his original art studio into a woodworking workshop and started making acoustic guitars which, I was informed by his family, were beautiful instruments. On some of his visits to James he brought a guitar with him and played classical pieces, entertaining not only James but others in the park.

When I reflect on those times now with decades of life, professional and academic experience, I can recognise in Gordon's behaviour the dichotomies that many people with severe mental illness – and those around them – experience: sensitivity and creativity, mixed with tormented thoughts and irrational actions.

Gordon had progressed through life to death from an intelligent, talented and creative person to a tortured soul.

The following year after Gordon's death, I thought that it might soon be time for James and I to spread our wings and leave the safety of the nest that Mum and Dad had created for us.

I enrolled in a Master of Health Science at Queensland University of Technology (QUT) so that I would be better qualified to take up a position as a nurse educator and be able to leave shift work as a clinical nurse. I left Tweed Heads Private Hospital and started working at the Gold Coast Hospital (GCH), teaching the last cohort of student nurses trained in the old apprenticeship system. Two evenings a week I drove up to QUT to attend lectures. On those days, I left home from Banora Point at 7:30am to get to GCH to teach and finally arrived home later that evening – around 9pm – after a two-hour drive from Brisbane.

They were long, exhausting days but worth the tiredness for the stimulation of learning and discovery of new ways of thinking, not to mention the security of knowing James was being well cared for by Mum and Dad.

At the end of that year, I successfully applied for a position as a lecturer at Griffith University's new School of Nursing at the Gold Coast campus, created in response to the shift from hospital-based training to university education for nurses. Thinking back to that time, I must have been overly optimistic about my capacity to cope with many changes because, in addition to starting a new job and continuing my postgraduate studies, I bought a house 45-minutes drive north of my parents which necessitated transferring James to a new school and finding after-school care.

I had spent considerable time researching primary schools that had a Special Education Unit (SEU) close to the university and found one with consistently good reviews from parents, so then looked for houses in the catchment area of that school.

Bingo!

I found a lovely town house in Highland Park, on the Gold Coast, with views to the hinterland and within walking distance of William

Duncan Primary School. Next came the daunting task of finding suitable after-school care for James.

I believe through God's providence I was led to looking in the local paper. There, I found a notice from a couple with prior experience in fostering children with special needs now offering to provide support to a school aged child in their locality. My phone call to them revealed that they lived around the corner from our new home and were not at all perturbed about catering to James' needs. John ran his own business from home and Barbara agreed to pick James up from school each day and look after him till I picked him up – which on my two study days wasn't until 8pm.

James and I moved into our new house and on the very first night I was confronted by a very large huntsman spider on the wall of my bedroom. Shock, horror! *What will I do?*

Ring Dad, of course, who can solve any problem.

He responded with 'and what do you want me to do?'

Oh dear, here I was 39 years old having left the nest for a second time and trembling at the thought of dealing with a spider on my own.

Just get on with it!

Barbara (or Mrs B, as James affectionately called her) went above and beyond physical care of James. She taught him to do French Knitting to keep his fingers occupied when he started skin picking – a common characteristic of PWS – and she introduced us to Gold Coast Recreation and Sport (GCRS), an organisation set up to provide support and services to children and adults with disabilities. In the years ahead, James enjoyed Special Olympics soccer and basketball through this organisation.

Once settled into the new house, school and job, it was very important to me to find a local church were James and I would be welcomed. After a few visits to various churches in the area, we found our spiritual home at Nerang Uniting Church and soon bonded with members of the congregation, some who ended up becoming long-term close friends.

James loved attending Sunday School, which continued his Christian journey that he had started with his Nanna many years before reading children's Bible stories first thing in the morning. Another aspect of James' journey was attending Christian-led holiday camps run by the Uniting Church. Not only did James grow spiritually, emotionally and socially attending these camps, but he had a profound effect on others with him.

The following is an extract of a letter from one of those impacted by James:

> *Dear Liz,*
>
> *My name is Jason and I was on a MAX Camp at Tallebudgera with your son James earlier this year. I have been meaning to write to you since that camp to share with you what an impact your son had on me and many others since that camp.*
>
> *I was James' carer and I found this to be challenging and rewarding. I also learnt a lot about servanthood and what it truly means to be a Christian… James showed me and we talked a lot about what we as Christians are called to do. I want to share with you an experience I had on camp with your son.*
>
> *We were in the change rooms talking and James asked me 'Jason, how many people in our small group are Christians?' I said a couple of them didn't know Jesus and weren't involved in the church. James replied, 'we need to tell them so when Jesus comes back to earth, they are ready'. I asked James what was going to happen when Jesus comes back and he replied 'he is going to heal my disability'.*

Despite his physical and mental disabilities, James knows Jesus in such an intimate way that I have rarely seen. I have since shared that experience with many people in my church and other friends and they have all been deeply moved.

I know James will continue to touch many people over the course of his life. I thank God for him and the opportunity I had to share this time with James.

God bless,

Jason

James' intimate relationship with Jesus was further revealed some time later when he was very unwell. James and I had contracted a particularly nasty bug whilst en route to Melbourne to spend holidays with my sister Sue. We both had severe gastroenteritis, resulting in me being hospitalised while Sue cared for James at home. She asked James to roll onto his side in bed so she could place a towel under him. He responded 'I can't, Jesus is lying there.'

During our second year at Highland Park, new neighbours arrived in the town house next door. After our first meeting sharing morning tea together, my next experience of Judy and Graham involved Graham tipping a bucket of water on my head from the balcony above. Ever the practical joker, Graham thought it would be a good way of testing my sense of humour! I must have passed the test because we became firm, lifelong friends. Judy rescued me many times from hours of James screaming in emotional distress and, in turn, having overcome my fear of huntsman spiders, I rescued her from infestations of spiders in her house when Graham was away on business.

Initiated by Gordon's death, James and I had left the security and familiarity of home life with Mum and Dad, support from the North

Coast Family Support Group and fellowship with our local Christian tribe in Tweed Heads to start another phase of our lives.

Perhaps we weren't actually flying yet, but optimistically flapping our wings with God providing the updraft!

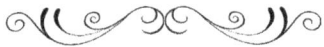

Confronting the Boundaries

Negotiating the continuum of inclusive education

It is 1995 and I am sitting in a Parents and Citizens meeting at Merrimac State High School on the Gold Coast, next to another mother Lyn whose son, like James, was enrolled in the Special Education Unit (SEU) of this school. The meeting had been convened to discuss issues that Lyn and I had raised about the lack of inclusion of our sons in any mainstream activities of the school. The discussion had not long started when a teacher from the mainstream section of the school proclaimed in a very loud and angry voice, 'we have enough kids to deal with in our classes who are not quite thick enough to be in the SEU without having to deal with your lot!'

But as for you, teach what accords with sound doctrine.
Titus 2:1

Needless to say, Lyn and I were shocked by this public outburst from a teacher, but not surprised by the expressed sentiment. Both of us had been subject to rejection of any proposal we had put forward to the school to have our sons included for a few hours per week in mainstream classes. This situation was in sharp contrast to what they had experienced at primary school.

James and Lyn's son had spent the previous four years at William Duncan Primary School, well integrated in mainstream classrooms while being ably supported by Special Education Unit staff who provided assistance to both students and mainstream teachers when required. It was an exemplar model of inclusive education where students with special needs were not only included, but welcomed in all activities with their peers.

James thrived at that school, keeping up academically and (mostly) enthusiastically engaged in learning. Thanks to the Special Education Unit staff who wanted to understand all they could about Prader-Willi Syndrome and its inherent challenging behaviours, his emotional meltdowns were handled competently and sensitively.

People with PWS have a number of underlying issues that cause them to have meltdowns. Most are highly anxious all the time. They have trouble regulating their emotions, and meltdowns can occur when they experience an unexpected change to routine or disappointment. Their anxiety often results in behaviours characterised by avoidance, non-compliance, perseveration, argumentativeness, verbal and / or physical aggression. This tendency towards meltdowns separates PWS from other developmental disabilities and can be very difficult to manage.

During the final year at William Duncan School, parents of children linked with the Special Education Unit were invited to attend information sessions about secondary school options. There were not many – the high school in our catchment area, a Special School and one high school with a new Special Education Unit a few suburbs away.

At that time, enrolment in a Special School was dictated by level of intellectual disability and because James' IQ was assessed as borderline, he did not immediately qualify. That didn't bother me. I assumed – wrongly – that a secondary school Special Education Unit would operate in the same way that we had experienced at William Duncan. I quite happily and confidently enrolled James at Merrimac, the high school with the new Unit, knowing that the mainstream high school in our area had large classes and no provision for students with special learning needs.

My confidence was short-lived. The Special Education Unit was situated in a building at some distance from the rest of the school buildings. It accommodated 10 students, one teacher and their aide. It was a school room decked out like a kindergarten. At recess times, students were contained within its confines. After initially being told that students in the Special Education Unit would have options to join some mainstream classes, those opportunities were not forthcoming.

The teacher was a friendly lady who, I believe, had the best intentions towards her students. However, it soon became evident to me that, while she was equipped to teach students with borderline to mild intellectual disabilities, she was struggling to manage challenging behaviours associated with various disabling conditions. James started having frequent behavioural outbursts. Each time, I was phoned at work and asked to take him home. I was told that the school did not have additional teacher aides to calm, distract or engage him when agitated.

Having seen what James could achieve with appropriate support, I was devastated to see him so distressed at school and I believed that, in part, this was due to boredom and a lack of behaviour management planning. I also thought that having only one teacher and one aide was not sufficient to adequately teach 10 students, each with special learning needs and unique behavioural challenges. My disappointment and frustration at attempts to engage with the school principal to discuss strategies to better support James and the Special Education Unit teacher soon turned to anger when it was suggested that I was interfering in school processes.

After being valued for my input to James' learning needs at all three of his primary schools, I naively assumed it would be the same in the secondary sector.

Not so!

I was ignored, dismissed, criticised and eventually ostracised. This was my first experience of the repercussions of advocacy.

I believe this happened because Lyn and I had been interviewed by a reporter from a local newspaper who had been alerted to an investigation by the Education Department into the operation of the Special Education Unit and the school's inclusion policy. This investigation was instigated by the Queensland Department of Education's South Coast region after Lyn and I had written to the regional director about the school's failure to implement the Department's social justice policy for inclusive education.

While this testing time was going on with the Department of Education, I was also under a lot of pressure at work. Our very small foundational team of lecturers at Griffith University was responsible for reviewing, upgrading and implementing the Bachelor of Nursing in line with new accreditation standards from the Queensland Nursing Council. In addition, we had to meet the academic expectations of the university – to publish or perish!

After several days of having to leave work early to pick up James from school and then settle him, I awoke one morning to the thought 'I can't do this anymore… I'm going to have a nervous breakdown.'

However, after a quick reckoning of my options I replaced that thought with 'not today, too much to do!'

Having only just survived two terms of James being at this school and with no positive changes in sight, I reluctantly transferred him to Southport Special School. It catered to students with a range of intellectual, physical and sensory disabilities, and had teacher to student ratios appropriate to the needs of the children. Despite my initial misgivings, the move was a positive one for James. He enjoyed a variety of learning experiences and, although he was probably not as cognitively stimulated as he was at primary school, he gained social skills and made friends.

Within a year at Southport Special School, James was attending Southport High School drama and art classes with a teacher aide to support him. Those experiences were the highlights of his week and he proudly brought home many wonderful works of art, including ceramics that he painted and fired himself. I still have some of them adorning my balcony.

In his final year at Southport Special School, James started employment experience in the Sheraton Mirage Hotel – working in their laundry. This was a really good fit for James. It involved predictable, routine activities working alongside mainly immigrants who accepted his differences just as they accommodated each other's. They provided clear instructions for him to follow and jobs that he could accomplish with minimal support. This work experience was so successful that the hotel offered him part-time work after leaving school, which continued for several years until severe mental illness intervened and curtailed his ability to be employed.

During James' post-primary school years, I completed the Master of Health Science, majoring in two areas: primary health care and education. Interestingly, my studies exposed me to the frameworks, conditions and practices of inclusive education – a basic human right – whether that be in a school or health-related setting. My lived experience – as a parent, university student, university academic and advocate – of inclusive education revealed a wide continuum of attitudes, commitment and understanding of the concept.

William Duncan Primary School demonstrated a good understanding of, and commitment to, the principles and practices of inclusive education. In stark contrast, failure to provide reasonable adjustments and targeted evidence-based support to James in his first experience of secondary schooling revealed how mismatched the reality was from the rhetoric of inclusive education in that environment. At another point on the continuum, Southport Special School – although only enrolling students with disabilities – offered them opportunities to learn and socialise with students at the nearby high school.

Although the education system today has made considerable progress towards inclusive education, the recent *Royal Commission into Violence, Abuse, Neglect and Exploitation of People with Disability* revealed that in schools of all types – mainstream, special and alternative – some students with disability are nevertheless enduring instances of harmful or inappropriate practices.

There is still much to do.

I am left wondering if the outspoken teacher in 1995 was a perpetrator of the segregation of students with disabilities, or perhaps a victim of an education system that did not adequately train and support its teachers to accommodate them.

Advocating for James' human right to be educated in an inclusive school setting was costly to my emotional wellbeing, but I have no regrets. I didn't knock down the boundaries, but I did contribute to an investigation by the Department of Education which resulted in an Internal School Review at Merrimac that brought some positive reforms in the following years.

My resilience to keep challenging the injustice was bolstered by having another parent stand shoulder to shoulder with me.

Unforeseen Blessings

The gift of allies on our path

It is a beautiful spring morning in 1999. I am travelling in a car with my friend Ruth on our way to a camp site in Hervey Bay, via Brisbane, to pick up her elderly father from his retirement home. We are towing a trailer packed with suitcases which belong to our Bethany Care group of people travelling by train to the same destination. Nearing Brisbane, Ruth casually remarks, 'by the way, I've never driven with a trailer before and have no idea how to reverse it, but it will all be okay.'

Not for the first time, I am both awed and nervous at Ruth's bravado.

I thank my God for you every time I think of you.
Philippians 1:3

A few years previously, I had encountered Ruth at Nerang Bowl where James and I had been guided by Gold Coast Recreation and Sport to find a 10-pin bowling group for people with disabilities. The group was run by Bethany Care, an organisation founded by Ruth and her husband many years before. They had started this very small home-based organisation to provide support to people with complex disabilities, including their son Nathan.

Sadly, Ruth's husband died not long after, but fortunately her church – Hope Christian Church – brought Bethany Care in under its auspice. Soon, she had volunteers from the church to assist her with the bowling group and a few other recreational activities. After a week or two of meeting Ruth, she proclaimed very confidently, 'I've been asking God for another Director to join Bethany Care, and I think he has sent you!'

I was initially stunned into silence, thinking *oh dear, what have I gotten myself into!*

Eventually, I responded that I would pray about it. I did, and I met with her pastor, and I said yes.

Our first foray into taking the Bethany bowling group on a short holiday was to a local camp site on the Gold Coast. By this time, I had recruited Robert from my church as a volunteer with Bethany Care – in much the same way as Ruth recruited me. He had been transporting people with disabilities living in supported accommodation to church on Sundays, and other church run social activities. We invited them to come with the Bethany group to camp.

With great confidence and faith in our ability to meet the needs of our fellow campers, we set off. Like me, Ruth was a registered nurse and we both had a very pragmatic approach to life, while weighing up the benefits and risks of our intended activities. We all survived with no mishaps and had great fun. With a few other successes like that under our belt, we planned the Hervey Bay trip to take the group whale watching.

Ruth managed to drive the car and trailer down the long driveway to her father's unit in Brisbane and, as she had faithfully predicted, at the right time and in the right place there was someone – the gardener – at the end of the driveway to guide the reversal back out. We, and all the train travelers, made it safely to Hervey Bay and back to the Gold Coast after a few days of sightseeing and sailing alongside several whales – what an awe-inspiring experience that was!

One of our Bethany Care travelers, David, had a penchant for slapping people on the back when he got excited. It didn't matter who it was, but whenever he sighted a whale, the nearest person got an enthusiastic whack with a great exclamation from David – 'there she blows!'

Fortunately, our fellow whale watching companions from the general public were either bemused and tolerant of such exuberance, or kept their distance!

Just like Jason, who acknowledged how much he had learnt about servanthood from his time looking after James at MAX Camp, I too had my portions of patience, tolerance and compassion increased while caring for our Bethany Care travelers. Each person was disabled in a different way and had their own unique needs, but all responded positively to simple kindness and respect. They ministered to our souls just as much as we ministered to their physical needs. Unbridled laughter became our common language. The look of wonder and amazement on their faces during our traveling activities also spoke volumes.

Interestingly, one of my agnostic friends, Denise, who had recently been diagnosed with terminal cancer and was staying with me while recuperating from treatment, confided that she could see the face of God in some of our Bethany Care recipients. She had come with me and James to a Saturday morning bowling group and sat with a couple of bowlers while they waited their turn. Two were non-verbal and just sat either side of Denise holding her hands and smiling.

She later told me that this had been a spiritual experience for her – something she had not previously encountered and couldn't easily put into words. She just felt at peace. Just before Denise died, some months later, she asked me, 'is it too late for God to accept me?'

What a privilege it was to say, 'it is never too late.'

Throughout the New Testament of the Bible, there are accounts of Jesus advising his followers to have a childlike humble and trusting attitude towards entering the kingdom of God – no expectation that power, good works, money or reputation is required. I wonder if Denise's spiritual experience opened not only her eyes, but her heart to this revelation?

As presented in previous chapters, James and I have had many blessed encounters – some lasting a short time, perhaps a few years, while others have been ongoing.

Joan, from the Shepherd Centre for hearing impaired children, came into our lives when I was feeling lost and helpless. She was bright, positive and encouraging – teaching James and me to discern and appreciate the beauty of sounds from nature while encouraging James to express himself vocally.

Judith, from the Early Intervention Teaching Program, brought compassion and perseverance to every facet of her interactions with James. Perhaps, having the lived experience of a sister with Down Syndrome gave her the ability to empathise with families' fears and expectations of the world beyond the acceptance, safety and security of the early intervention enclave. Judith became both teacher and confidante.

Jason, the carer on the Uniting Church MAX Camp, in his very brief encounter with James was so impacted by his unquestioning faith that Jesus would one day return and heal him, that he continued to relate this story many years later to friends and congregations. I managed to locate and communicate with Jason 30 years after that camp experience and he still remembered James.

Barbara and John, unable to have children of their own, provided for the special needs of other people's children. Caring for a child with Prader-Willi Syndrome can be a daunting experience even for the most loving of parents, but Barbara met this challenge head on when she offered to care for James after school. Calm and practical, Barbara found creative ways to address some of James' anxiety-driven behaviours while enabling me to work and study without fear of unexpected calls to retrieve him.

Judy and Graham brought more than just 'nice neighbours' with them when they moved in next door. They became extended family, enjoying the good times with us and digging in when things got really tough. No matter what Judy was doing, she would respond immediately to my frequent and frantic cries for help when James was having endless meltdowns. We were never excluded from their social events, despite James' difficult behaviours.

While we were neighbours, Judy and Graham attended a few of our church social activities but were not regular church-goers. Both had some church experiences during childhood but, while not dismissing the existence of God, neither had a personal and committed faith. Unfortunately for us, they decided to move back to Adelaide where their children and grandchildren lived. We kept in regular contact. About a year after they returned to Adelaide, they told me that they had both embraced the Christian faith and were attending Aberfoyle Uniting Church. My heart sang.

A few years later, another surprise – Judy told me that they had a new minister from Queensland and his name was Brant. Many years previously we had a minister at Nerang Uniting Church called Brant and he, and his wife Neva, were well known to us.

Could this be the same person?

Yes, it was!

In recent years, I have spent many holidays in Adelaide with Judy and Graham and a group of their church friends – Brant and Neva included. The connections kept growing.

Robert, a quiet soul from our church in Nerang who started volunteering with Bethany Care, went on to become one of their part-time paid workers after the organisation started receiving funding from the Queensland Government. He provided in-home care for James when I was required to attend interstate and international conferences for work. James felt safe and secure in Robert's care, which was a comfort to me. Robert's mission in life was to care deeply for others and he did just that with compassion and humility.

Not long after Judy and Graham moved to Adelaide, James and I moved a short distance away to a larger house with a yard so we could have a dog one day. Once again, our neighbours – Bette and Terry – became both friends and supporters to James. Bette offered to give James piano lessons after school, so several afternoons a week he went in next door and she taught him to read the notes and play simple tunes, eventually progressing to using both hands. It still amazes me how patient and encouraging she was. James loved his time with Bette.

Stepping out in faith can be scary and there have been times when I wondered if God was with us on this journey. Often, it has only been with hindsight that I have realised that the right people were in the right place just at the right time of need – they were allies on our path. God had provided, but maybe not in the ways I had been expecting.

Blessed encounters did not stop there. Skip forward to 2011.

After many discussions with my sister Sue, and much consideration of the upheaval of another move on James, my parents and myself, I decided that James and I would relocate from Queensland to Melbourne. I had completed a PhD and been promoted up the academic rankings to Professor while at Griffith University. I was ready for a change, and prayed that reports I had read, citing Victoria as a leader in disability care, would match reality.

Initially, James and I lived with my sister and her husband in Eltham while we were waiting for our house to be built in St Helena. James started attending Araluen Centre day services. He benefitted from acquiring new friends and having very experienced and committed instructors – all of them were great, but Kerryn and Cindy formed a very special bond with James. Even after leaving employment at Araluen, Kerryn continues to support James by taking him to Boxing Day Test Cricket matches.

Upon hearing that there was a Disability Expo about to be held at Broadmeadows, I decided to attend to find out what respite and / or holiday options might be available and suitable for James. After spending a couple of hours wandering between different provider stands and repeatedly being informed that their staff to client ratios were in the order of 1:8 or more, I gave up and headed for the exit. James needed high level support, and was used to being in small groups with very experienced support workers.

Just by the exit I was attracted to a very small stand staffed with just two people. Their poster read:

> 'Wow Tours – a boutique style day respite and short holiday service catering to individual preferences and capacities and supported by highly skilled staff.'

Fortunately, I had just enough determination left to stop. After a lengthy discussion with the founders, John and Kay, about James' needs, I left with a date and time that they would visit us at home to spend some time getting to know him. They came a week or so later, and there began a long and fruitful relationship of support and friendship.

After that day in 2011, James began his association with Wow Tours with day trips, swimming with the dolphins in Port Philip Bay, then progressed to short holidays within Victoria and later to longer holidays interstate. During the protracted Covid outbreak lockdowns, when day programs shut down, Wow Tours – now with a name change to Oassist – was given permission to take James on walks in local parks. What a life changer that was! Without that, James would have spent long, lonely days at home, ruminating on his anxieties.

In recent years, Oassist has sustained their exemplary care of James, facilitating community participation activities five and a half days a week with 1:1 support while continuing to provide short holiday breaks in small groups. Holidays back to the Gold Coast enabled James to visit his Nanna and Pa who had moved into residential aged care since we had relocated to Melbourne. John's son Josh – James' primary 1:1 support worker – accompanied James to the Gold Coast to attend his Pa's 100th birthday along with me and all the extended family and friends. Having attended that celebration, James' 40th birthday party and other social group activities, John, Kay and Josh have become 'adopted' members of the family.

James and I have been truly blessed by so many people who have travelled with, and supported, us on our journey of life with disability and mental illness.

Could this be God's providence?

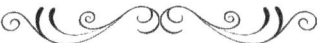

Passport to Possibilities

Experiencing the joys and jitters of traveling

It is 13 February 2004 and I am sitting in the restaurant of the Radisson Hotel in Los Angeles, USA with my sister Sue and James. We are exhausted after a long flight from Australia. A waiter appears with our meals – each plate piled high with enough food to feed an army! Sue and I look at each other in utter dismay while James' eyes nearly pop out with anticipation of a feast.

Oh dear, what have we gotten ourselves into?

Removing any food from James' plate will cause a meltdown and we don't want that on our first night in America. Sixteen more days of our vacation to go.

Can we survive to tell the tale?

So do not worry about tomorrow; it will have enough worries of its own. There is no need to add to the troubles each day brings.
Matthew 6:34

Over the past 20 years, Sue and I have often recalled this vacation with amazement and hilarity. We did survive and we all enjoyed some wonderful sights and experiences – but, not without some hairy moments.

Previous holidays with James had all been within Australia and staying with family or friends who were well versed in the 'Prader-Willi lifestyle' – that is, predictable meal times, appropriate food choices and portions, and structured activities that James could cope with. Everything was planned with an expectation that an event might have to be changed at the last minute if he was not having a good day. Even with contingencies in place, these holidays were often fraught with unanticipated hiccups.

What were we thinking of when we decided to take James overseas to fulfill his desire to go to Disneyland?

I'm not sure really, other than perhaps having some idea that Sue and I had the strength and capacity to cope with whatever lay ahead of us. More important than that though was my determination to give James the opportunity to experience something that a lot of people his age would take for granted.

After a bit of web surfing, I found a holiday advertised as the 'Best of the West' incorporating a coach trip – with booked accommodation – starting and finishing in Los Angeles and touring through Santa Monica, Santa Barbara, Santa Maria, Monterey, San Francisco, Yosemite Valley, Fresno, Bakersfield, Las Vegas, the Grand Canyon, Sedona, Phoenix, Yuma and San Diego.

James had often said he would love to go to Disneyland and Universal Studios, so signing up for the Best of the West trip presented an opportunity to grant his wish and to see a selection of America's cities, towns, tourist attractions and landscapes.

When I first mentioned my plans to Sue, I expected her response to be along the lines of, 'have you lost your mind?'

Instead, she said, 'how about I come with you?'

So, on the 13th of February 2004, the three of us took off from Sydney airport on a direct flight to Los Angeles and arrived some 15 hours later. We were very fortunate to have spare seats next to us so James lay down and slept most of the way. The beauty of going on an organised trip was being picked up from the airport and taken straight to the hotel.

So far, so good – until it was time to think about dinner.

Not wanting to stray too far from the hotel on our first night, we thought the hotel restaurant would be a good option. Bad decision. We had no prior experience of restaurant meal sizes in America and couldn't believe our eyes when we saw the plates.

It was not a Prader-Willi friendly experience at all, but we got through that night without a major incident. James was too tired to notice our surreptitious removal of half his plate contents which remained well hidden in napkins under the table.

Lesson well learnt!

We did some research about other eating options, and for the remainder of the trip headed straight for Subway at lunchtimes and Hometown Buffet for dinner. Thankfully, nearly every place we stopped at on the coach trip had a Hometown Buffet, or equivalent family buffet-style restaurant, so we could select appropriate food for James in the right portions. It got a bit boring for Sue and I, but that didn't matter because it lessened everyone's anxiety.

The first two days of the tour were free from scheduling and Disneyland was an easy walk from the Radisson Hotel so we could take our time to explore all the amazing attractions. James loved it, but was a bit taken aback when larger-than-life Disney characters approached him for a chat and photo opportunity. We availed ourselves of assistance provided to persons with a disability – picking up a wheelchair when there was going to be a long walk and dense crowds – so we were often taken to the front of the queue for admission to theaters and arenas.

Sometimes, being with a disabled person has its advantages!

Meeting our fellow coach travelers for the first time revealed many other Australians and a few New Zealanders, so we felt quite at home. After a day at Universal Studios and a tour around Hollywood, off we set up the western coastline, stopping at some beautiful beaches along the way – perhaps not quite as beautiful as our beaches, though!

Only a few days into the trip, James started looking quite unwell; pale and glassy-eyed. We soon discovered why when the gastro signs appeared. Yuck! It was not a pleasant experience on board a bus with one toilet. Fortunately, we soon arrived in San Francisco where we had a two-night stay and friends from Australia living there. One was a doctor (albeit a psychiatrist) but he still remembered his basic medical training and brought us some medication to ease some of James' symptoms.

One of our sightseeing experiences while in San Francisco was a ferry ride to Alcatraz Island and a tour of the old prison relics. James did not enjoy that day at all; partly still feeling unwell but, we were later to find out, very traumatised by the stories told of prison life, particularly references to deprivation of food.

To this day, James suffers from a terrifying delusion of being locked up in prison and starved.

Although he was feeling much better on the morning of departure from San Francisco, James decided he wasn't going to get out of the bath and our attempts to extract him only resulted in loud screaming. Our second big hurdle of the trip to get over – the coach was about to arrive and we couldn't hold everybody up.

Mercifully for us, our wonderful coach driver Josephine and tour guide Lisa were very understanding and waited while we eventually cajoled James out of the bath, into his clothes and onto the bus, where he promptly fell asleep. Ever since toddlerhood, James could usually be eased out of a meltdown and into a calm sleep by being driven around in a car. The same effect was happening in the coach.

It has only been in recent times that sensory assessments undertaken by an Occupational Therapist has identified motion as a primary modulator for James' emotional regulation – very common for people with 'autistic-like' characteristics.

Perhaps my choice of going on a coach tour wasn't so crazy after all!

Although it was over 20 years ago, I vividly recall the awe-inspiring scenery we drove through, and the fun we had with our driver, guide and fellow travelers. Yosemite Valley National Park stands out as one of these unforgettable experiences; all sorts of animals roaming freely among the woodlands of the valley, surrounded by majestic snow-capped mountains. Josephine, the coach driver, was obviously very experienced at hiding behind the coach and bombarding returning travelers with snow balls – she didn't miss any of us!

It was so good to see James laughing and joining in the frivolity.

From the snow in Yosemite, we headed south-east through Fresno's agricultural landscape in the heart of California's Central Valley to Bakersfield, birthplace of the country music genre – Bakersfield Sound – then across the arid Mojave Desert to Las Vegas. Sue and I loved seeing the changing landscapes from the comfort of our coach and hearing Lisa's commentary about the history of the places we were driving through, while James snoozed on.

We stayed in the Mirage Hotel in Las Vegas, home to Siegfried and Roy's Secret Garden and Dolphin Habitat. One of James' favourite pastimes has always been visiting zoos, animal sanctuaries and any shows highlighting animals so he was in his element. It was amazing to see the star attractions – white lions and tigers. Unfortunately, Siegfried and Roy's magic and illusion show in the Mirage casino had been discontinued the previous year after Roy was critically injured by one of the tigers during a performance.

We had our third hairy moment of the trip in Las Vegas. We had planned to go to the Fountains of Bellagio display where more than a thousand fountains sway in front of the hotel, enhanced by music and lighting. James was initially happy to go but, somehow in the middle of the vast foyer of the Bellagio Hotel, he got the jitters and expressed his anxiety with very loud remonstrations. Sue managed to keep concerned on-lookers away while I contained James and got him to a nearby chair to calm down. I think we must have been surrounded by angels because no security men came near us and James settled enough to see some of the fountain and lighting display.

Another near miss, but we adapted and survived.

Leaving Las Vegas, we headed north-east to Zion National Park surrounded by massive sandstone cliffs of cream, pink and red. A stop at a lookout revealed the long narrow Zion Canyon, cut out by the Virgin River. Traveling through Mount Carmel Junction we headed north to Bryce Canyon where we stayed overnight at Ruby's Inn surrounded by deep snow.

Once again, Josephine ambushed us with snowballs as we alighted from the coach. Together with Lisa, she also constructed a large snowman during the night just outside our motel door which greeted us when we emerged in the morning. We had formed some close bonds with our fellow travelers, particularly families with children so James was able to join in their fun of adding bits to the snowman while hurling giant snowballs at each other.

The most memorable scenery of Bryce Canyon was the Bryce Amphitheater, which was home to the largest concentration on earth of the crimson-colored, spire-shaped rock formations known as hoodoos. We stopped at a few viewpoints around the amphitheater to see different aspects of the hoodoos. What an awe-inspiring experience that was!

From there, we re-traced our journey back through Mount Carmel south-east and skirted the rim of the Grand Canyon to its southern border. It was here that joy and jitters merged when I bravely decided to join a few others on a helicopter ride over the south rim of the Canyon. I had voiced both interest and fear about this opportunity to Sue as we neared the site of the Papillion Helicopters, and she convinced me that I would probably never get this chance again.

Because of passenger weight distribution, I got seated at the front next to the pilot. 20+ years later, I can vividly recall the helicopter skimming over the land and then suddenly it dropped away and we were soaring over the ginormous canyon. My stomach turned over a few times, as I clung to the handle in front with white knuckled hands. For someone who had always been scared of heights, this was above and beyond bravery – but breath-taking. I loved it. The photos I took nowhere near matched the bird's-eye views of the rock gorges, the Colorado River and Kaibab Forest lining the canyon's edge.

That was a once-in-a-lifetime experience.

It took a bit to come down off that 'high' and refocus on the next panoramas along the southward journey through Sedona to Phoenix. Along the way we saw the giant tree-like cacti Saguaro that towered above our heads – some taller than 12 meters! – along with the Montezuma Castle National Monument, a 20-room high-rise apartment built into a towering limestone cliff. This monument, built in 1906, is dedicated to preserving Native American culture and tells a story of ingenuity and survival in an unforgiving desert environment. Just south of Phoenix, we turned west to travel to our next major destination, San Diego.

On the way to San Diego, we passed through Yuma Territorial Prison State Historic Park where the old prison, built in 1876 and in operation for 33 years, is now a museum. Thankfully, we didn't stop to tour the museum because that would have just added to James' future fears and delusions about being imprisoned.

San Diego was our last stop before returning to Los Angeles, and we spent two days there exploring the beautiful beaches and parks. Once again, James got to indulge in one of his favourite activities when we visited the San Diego Zoo in Balboa Park. The best exhibit was the giant pandas. Another wonderful experience was sitting back on a harbour cruise, taking in the San Diego skyline, sailing under the Coronado Bridge and viewing the US Naval fleet and the harbour's resident sea lions.

All too soon, it was time to return to Los Angeles airport and wait for our flight back to Australia. Unfortunately for us, we were dropped at the airport six hours before our scheduled departure, so we spent a lot of time and energy trying to get comfortable enough for James to have a snooze. Thankfully, he coped without a meltdown.

Was the trip worth it?

Definitely! The many, many joys and wonderful experiences we had far outweighed the few jitters we endured along the way. Not only did we survive, but we were enriched.

Holding Together

Enduring the burden of deficiencies in mental health services

It is Christmas Day 2012 and I am sitting having lunch with my sister Sue, her family, Mum and Dad. I am breathing deeply, trying to swallow the huge lump in my throat and concentrate on the conversation but I can't hold it together. The dam bursts, the tears flow and I escape to the bedroom. I can't 'unsee' James restrained by the wrists and ankles on a bed in an Acute Psychiatric Unit and I can't 'unhear' his screams. Am I so disturbed because it is Christmas Day and the expectation is for peace, joy, love and hope? Probably, because this is not the first time this has happened. *Where are you God? Can you see what is happening? Can you hear him?*

> *Do not be afraid – I am with you!*
> *I will make you strong and help you:*
> *I will protect you and save you.*
> **Isaiah 4:10**

Since 2002, aged 21, James' demeanor and behaviour had escalated from the characteristic meltdowns of Prader-Willi Syndrome to the worrying signs of depression and psychosis – not uncommon in the syndrome, but worryingly similar to that manifested by his father before he died.

A meltdown is when a person with PWS is unable to control themselves due to heightened emotions. The behaviour that results can be anything from refusing to communicate or move, to uncontrollable screaming and crying – and in more extreme cases, self-harm, violence and recklessness.

In the 10 years preceding this hospital admission, James had been treated by five psychiatrists, had two emergency admissions to a psychiatric unit on the Gold Coast, had self-harmed twice, and had been prescribed nine different psychotropic medications – adversely reacting to four of them.

During this time, he had been given provisional diagnoses of major depressive disorder with psychotic features, generalised anxiety disorder with obsessional and compulsive features and post-traumatic stress disorder. However, none of the five psychiatrists could be conclusive in their diagnoses, because James' presentation did not closely match the usual diagnostic criteria for any of them.

Three psychiatrists, one in Queensland and two in Victoria, were associated with services for people with dual disability – intellectual and psychiatric – that provided second opinions to mainstream mental health services to clarify diagnoses and provide advice on treatment options. These services were not for ongoing psychiatric care unless there was high clinical need and the person was unable to access another appropriate provider. This was the case for James.

Finding a private psychiatrist willing to accept him as a patient was like looking for hens' teeth!

The other two psychiatrists were consultants in the public hospital where James had been admitted on the Gold Coast. Neither of them was familiar with Prader-Willi Syndrome, nor had any experience in treating people with intellectual disability.

Both of these admissions were via the Emergency Department and, in one case, James was not seen by a consultant psychiatrist for 48 hours. Instead, he was reviewed and treated by junior registrars resulting in being over-medicated and suffering acute buccolingual dystonia – an adverse reaction condition characterised by involuntary contractions of muscles of the face, neck, tongue and larynx. This was a terrifying experience for James and, to this day, when prescribed a new antipsychotic he will respond anxiously with, 'will it give me the tongue thing?'

Each time James had a meltdown in the ward – and there were many – he was manacled to the bed or put in seclusion. Medical and nursing staff admitted they did not know how to manage him because they had either no, or inadequate, training in complex behaviours associated with neurodevelopmental disabilities like PWS. Thankfully, the admissions were short because it became evident to all concerned that being in the psychiatric unit was more traumatising than therapeutic.

Fast forward to 2011, when James and I had moved to Melbourne. On referral from his GP, James was reviewed and treated for a short time by a psychiatrist from the Centre for Developmental Disability Health, and then by another psychiatrist from the Victorian Dual Disability Service. Both were compassionate, caring and competent practitioners. However, James' mental health continued to decline leading to an extremely traumatic transportation to hospital by paramedics and police on Christmas Eve of 2012.

Just like his previous admissions interstate, James was put in the high support area of the Acute Psychiatric Unit, accessed by two sets of internal locked doors. This area accommodated four patients, all highly volatile with the potential to harm themselves, other patients or staff. No doubt, it was a terrifying experience for any patient or visitor, but made worse for James being intellectually disabled and with pre-existing persecutory delusions of being arrested and locked up.

His delusions had become reality.

Despite being in a secure single room, every time he became verbally or physically aggressive a 'Code Grey' was called, defined as 'a response to occupational violence and aggression in Victorian public health services.' This resulted in at least two security personnel attending and restraining James, usually by securing his wrists and ankles to the bed frame while nursing staff administered fast acting medication in an effort to calm him. However, often the medication had little effect and he was kept physically restrained, sometimes for 20 minutes or more.

James was only 150 centimeters tall and weighed 49 kilograms, yet the physical restraint by two security officers continued. Safety of staff and patients is paramount but, for James, this short-term security protocol has resulted in long term post-traumatic stress.

As a registered nurse, I had seen physical restraint of patients many times. It is a very distressing experience for the patient, any relatives present and for the staff. Nobody likes witnessing physical aggression and I assume it is not a pleasant task for the security officers. Knowing all this doesn't help when you are the mother of the patient.

It is soul destroying.

As I write this chapter in 2025, I relive those three hospital admissions as well as four more in the acute psychiatric unit of a major Melbourne public hospital – one admission for six weeks and another for eight weeks. With each new admission, the staff became more familiar with James and the characteristics of Prader-Willi Syndrome, which greatly reduced the Code Grey calls. Nevertheless, he still spent most of his admissions in the high support area, partly because of the severity of his condition but also because there was no restriction of access to snack foods in the low support area of the ward.

This hospital has designated wards and staff for specific population groups or mental health conditions, for example:

- Child and Youth
- Adult
- Perinatal Parent and Infant
- Secure Extended Care
- Post Trauma Recovery
- Acquired Brain Injury
- Eating Disorders
- Neurological disease with mental illness

However, there is nothing specific to cater for people with developmental disability. Hence, patients like James are usually admitted to the acute adult psychiatric unit where there are no day-time activities appropriate to developmental level, and very few staff experienced in neuro-developmental disorders.

People with Prader-Willi Syndrome need predictable, structured routines with clear, concise and consistent communication. In an acute psychiatric unit, the only predictability is that staff will change constantly, patients will come and go, there will be frequent verbal and physical disturbances, there will be no routine times for medical examinations of patients and there will be inconsistent communication.

In this chaotic environment, James is at his most anxious.

When not in hospital, James spends every day in 1:1 supported, structured activities. He has a weekly calendar detailing who will be supporting him each day to access social and recreational activities in his local community. He relies on familiar people who can respond to his needs and can predict and plan for disruptions to expected routines. James still has high levels of anxiety even in this optimum environment.

That is why, during every admission, I have spent 8-10 hours per day in the ward with James struggling to keep him occupied while other patients attend individual and group therapy sessions not appropriate for him. It was mentally and emotionally exhausting. While individual nursing staff have been caring and receptive to wanting to understand more about Prader-Willi Syndrome and its unique characteristics, they have been constrained by time and competing demands on their attention.

Exacerbating this situation is the current bifurcated care across two siloed care systems – Health and the National Disability Insurance Scheme (NDIS). The Scheme may fund reasonable and necessary support to provide guidance and training for hospital staff working with participants who have challenging behaviours. However, while this may be possible for a planned admission, it is not feasible for emergency admissions. The NDIS will not typically fund support workers to help participants while they are in hospital, so it is left to families to provide accustomed support to their loved one.

Between hospital admissions, James' mental health care is managed by a public health continuing care service. He has a nurse case manager and is seen regularly by a consultant psychiatrist or registrar. Each of the psychiatrists or registrars who has reviewed him has been very attentive and responsive to information given to them by me and support workers, but the turnover is fairly frequent – there have been nine in eight years. This is not uncommon in the public mental health system.

Recently, a referral for admission to a psychiatric unit of a private hospital for James to have Transcranial Magnetic Stimulation treatment was refused because the hospital claimed they could not provide a sufficient level of nursing care for James. However, they suggested that he could have the treatment as a self-funded and self-supported outpatient. That disappointed, but did not surprise me.

The lack of integrated care options for individuals with intellectual disability and mental health conditions, system structural problems, professional training gaps and the need for a skilled workforce have been recognised by both the *Royal Commission into Violence, Abuse, Neglect and Exploitation of People with Disability* and *The Royal Commission into*

Victoria's Mental Health System. It was noted that the divide between health and disability sectors has left gaps in service provision and that responsibilities for caring for this vulnerable population group are vague, and not sufficiently funded.

As a mother and a person who spent my working career in healthcare, education and research, I think it is an indictment on our health and human services systems that low paid, certificate qualified, disability support workers are expected to provide complex physical and mental health support to people like James in a community setting 24 hours per day, yet degree qualified clinicians – in a controlled hospital environment – struggle with this responsibility.

Parents and carers, like me, are left to hope and pray that these deficiencies will be rectified and not used as political footballs to be kicked backwards and forwards between federal and state governments. Meanwhile we hold together the threads of formal care that are currently available and weave them with all the informal supports we can muster to support our loved ones with dual disability.

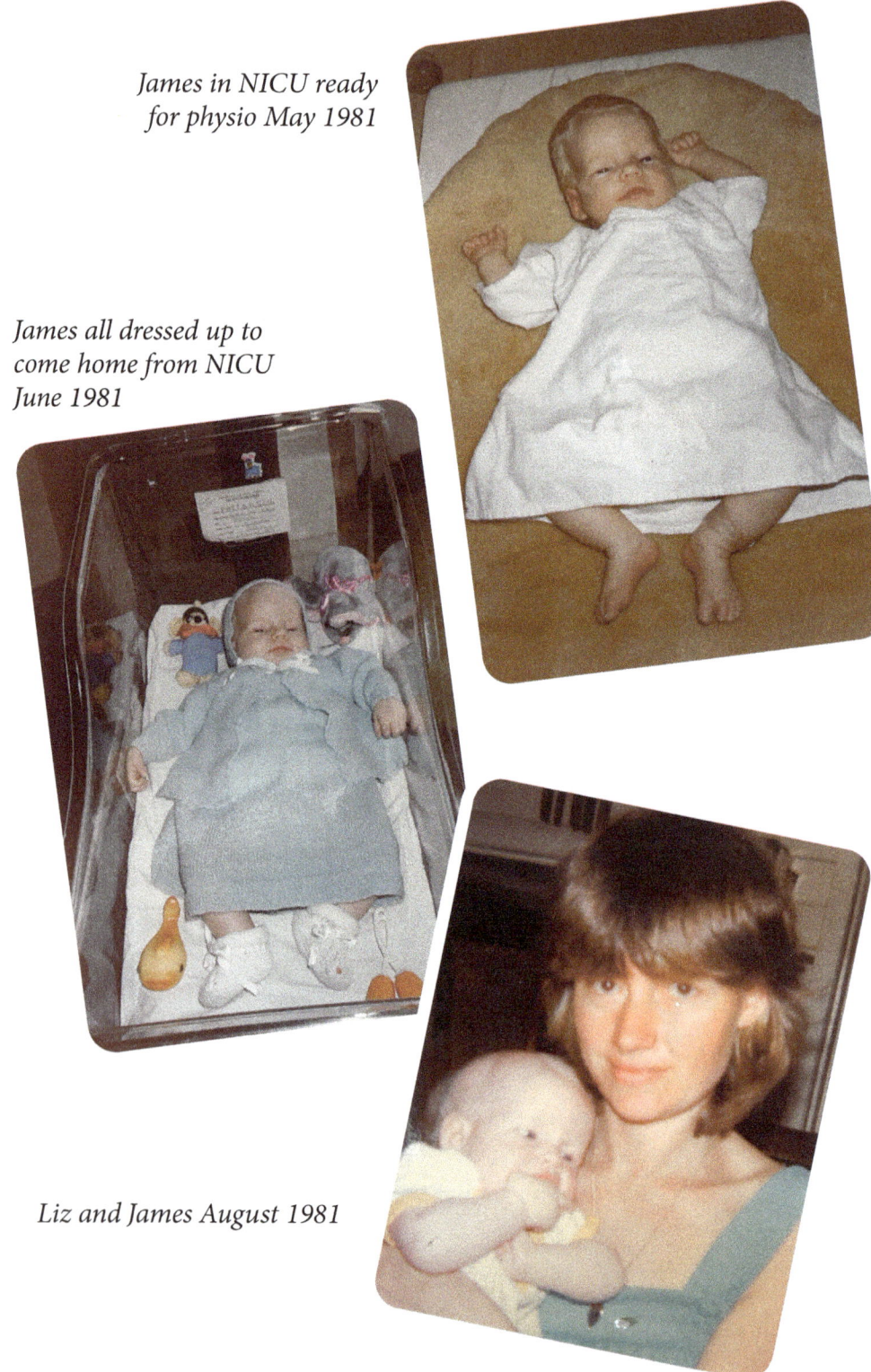

James in NICU ready for physio May 1981

James all dressed up to come home from NICU June 1981

Liz and James August 1981

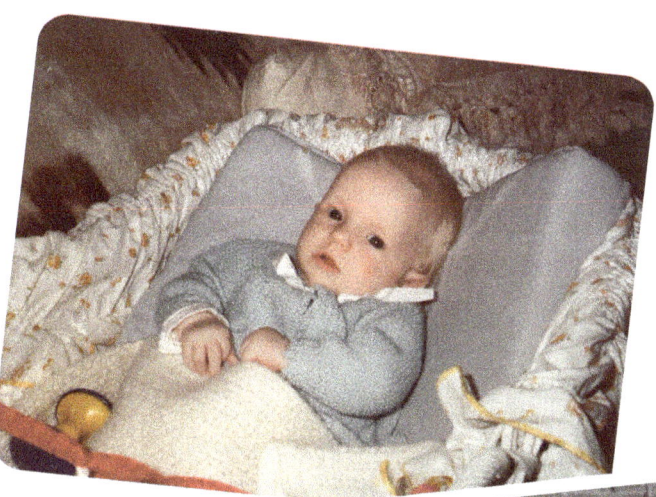

James enjoying a rest at Balmain September 1981

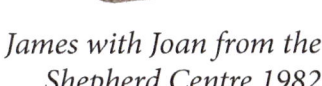

James with Joan from the Shepherd Centre 1982

Liz and James 1982

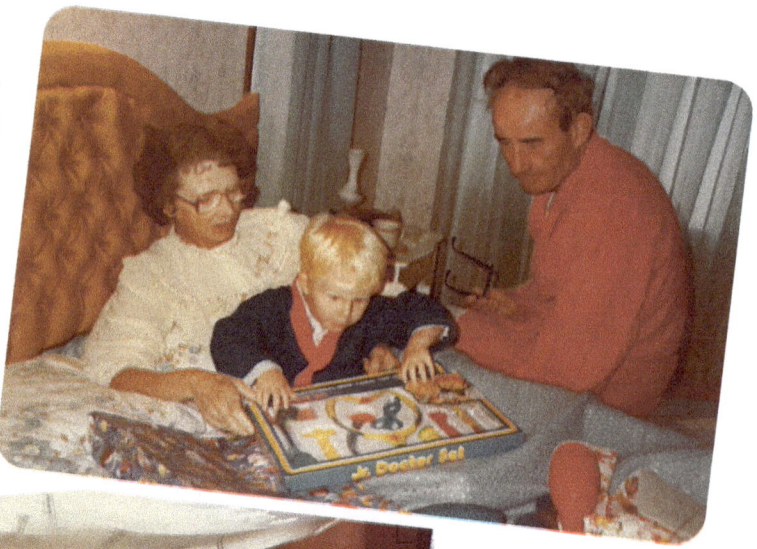

James with Nanna and Pa at Terranora 1984

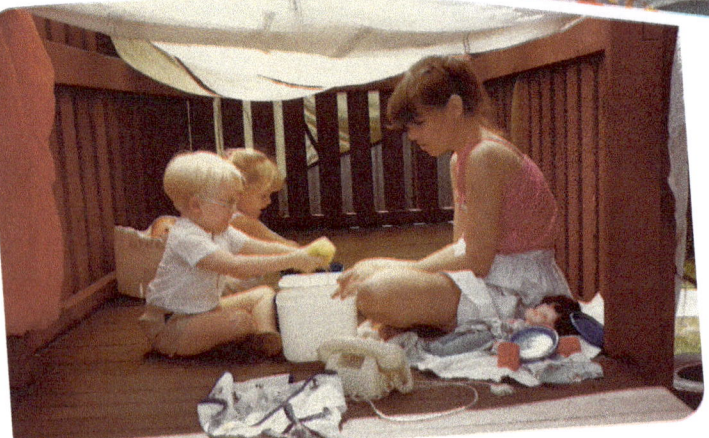

James with special teacher Judy at EITP 1984

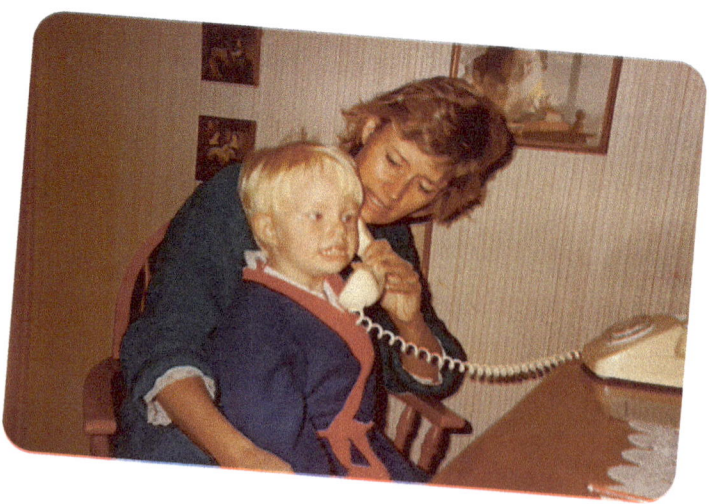

Liz and James at Terranora 1985

James with cousins Lee and Tim 1986

James' first day at Terranora Primary 1987

James with Nanna and Pa at Banora Point 1988

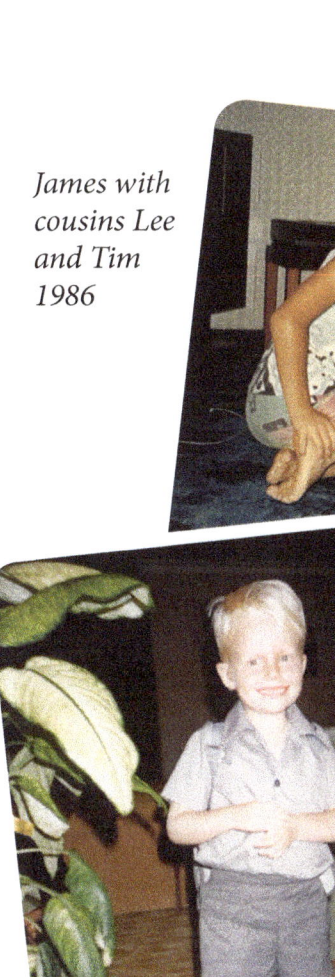

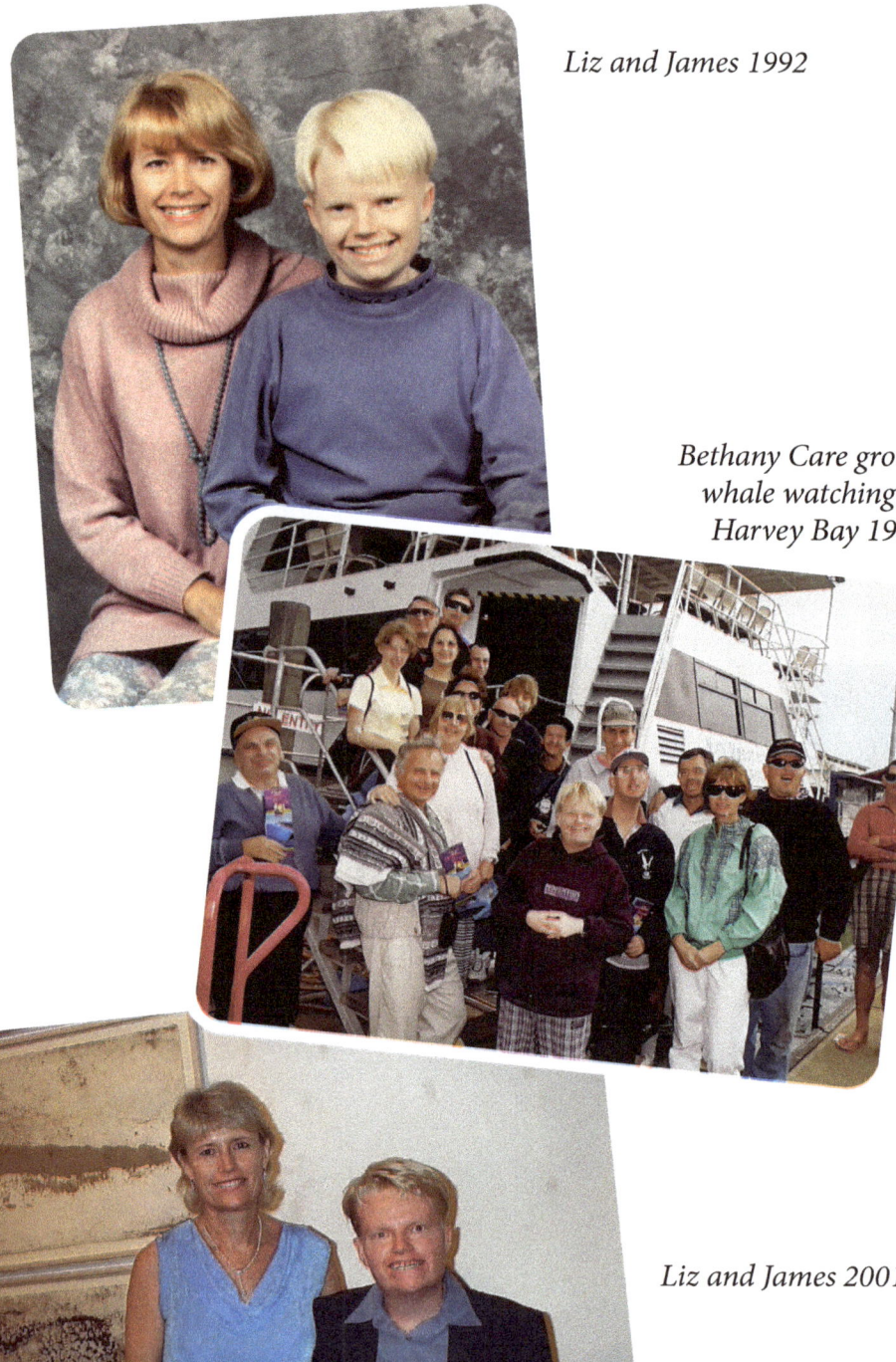

Liz and James 1992

Bethany Care group whale watching at Harvey Bay 1999

Liz and James 2001

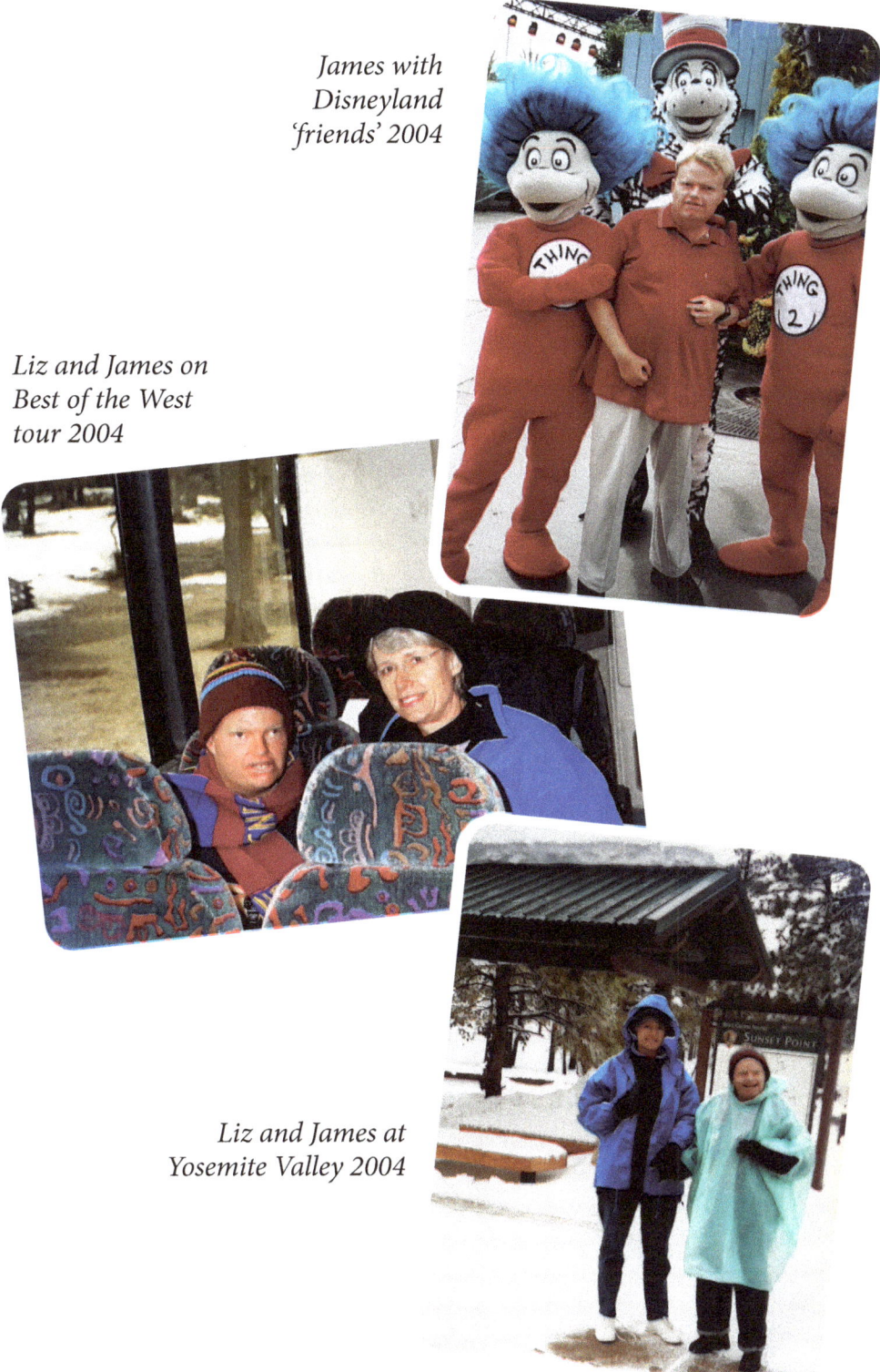

James with Disneyland 'friends' 2004

Liz and James on Best of the West tour 2004

Liz and James at Yosemite Valley 2004

James with Liz and Aunty Sue at Bryce Canyon 2004

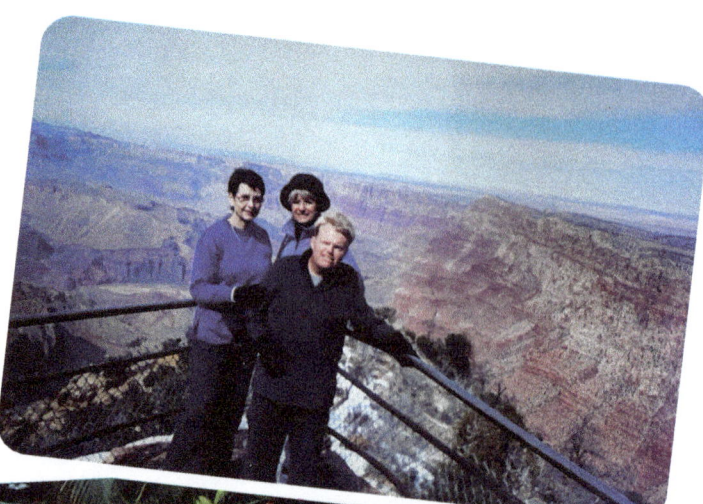

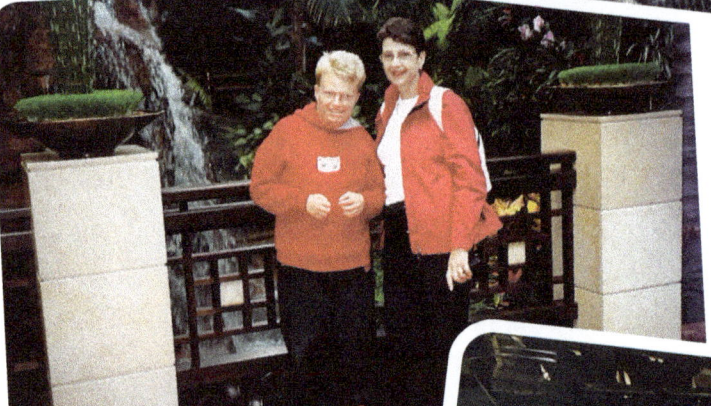

James with Aunty Sue at Las Vegas 2004

Liz and James at LA airport after Best of the West tour 2004

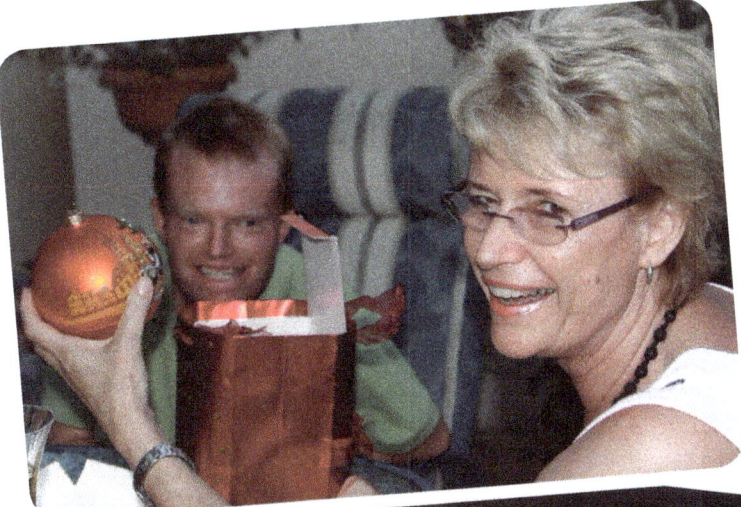

Liz and James Christmas 2008

James dancing at Wow Tours Rocks N Roll Trip 2016

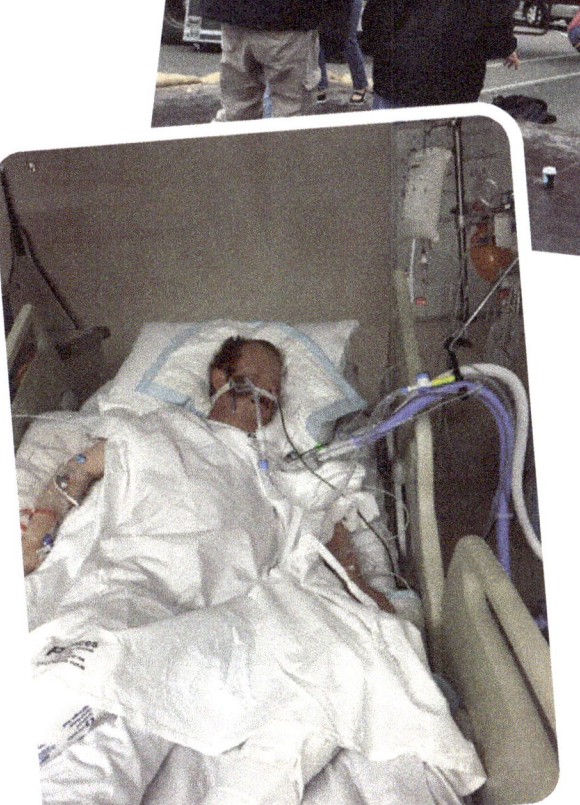

James in ICU after first emergency surgery March 2016

James at Eltham two weeks after ICU discharge 2016

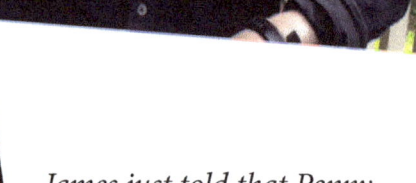
James just told that Penny belonged to him Nov 2016

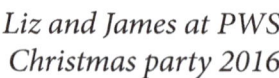
Liz and James at PWS Christmas party 2016

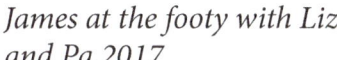
James at the footy with Liz and Pa 2017

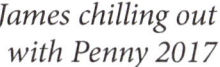
James chilling out with Penny 2017

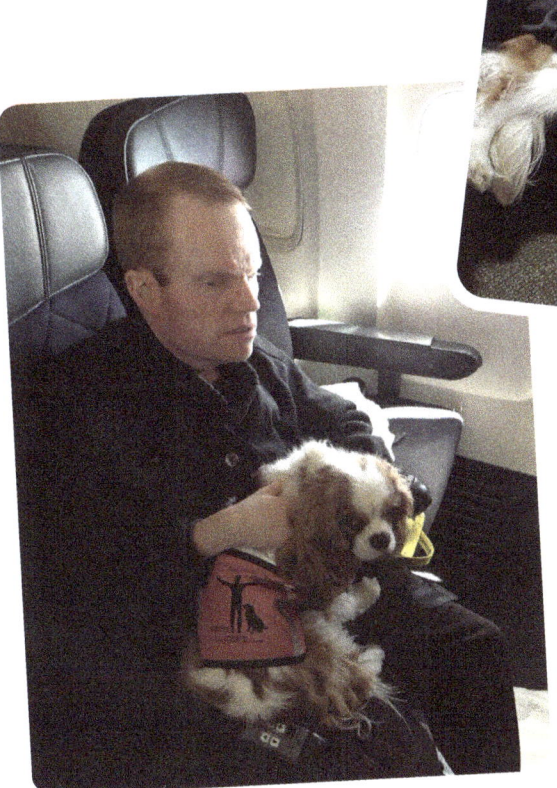
James and Penny on the plane going to the Gold Coast 2018

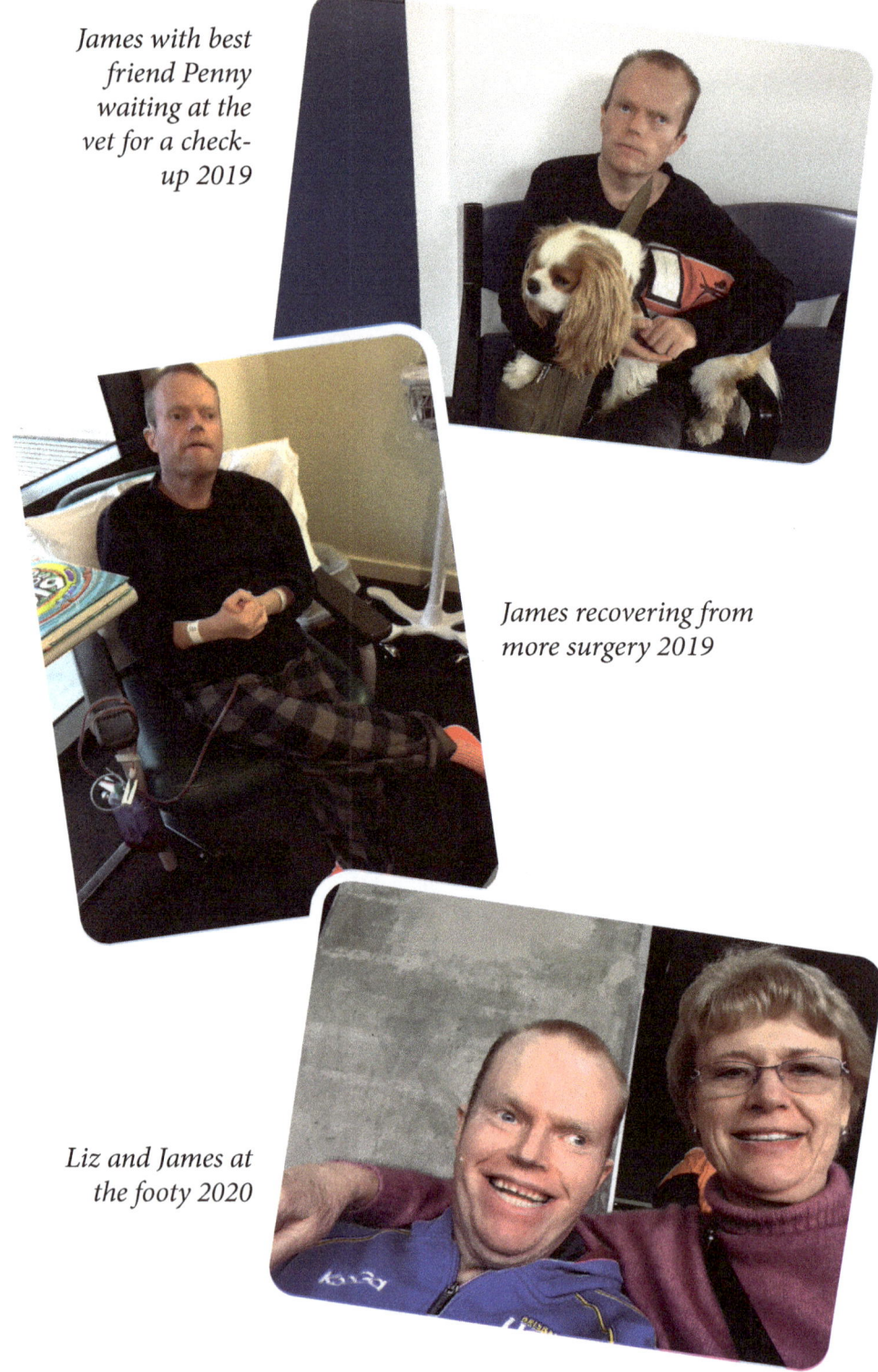

James with best friend Penny waiting at the vet for a check-up 2019

James recovering from more surgery 2019

Liz and James at the footy 2020

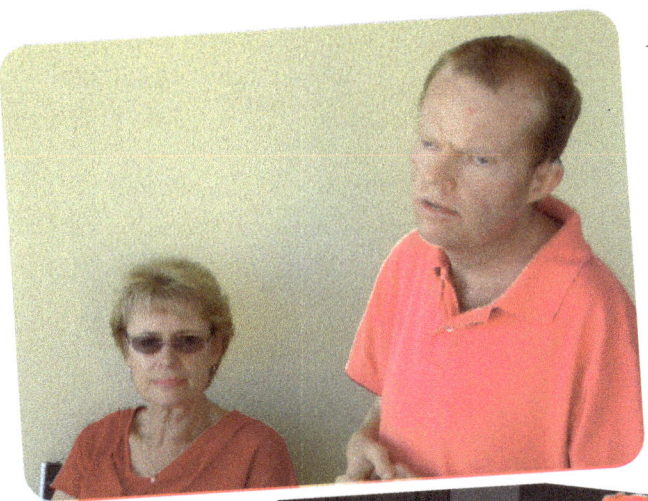

Liz and James 2020

James at Araluen Christmas party 2020

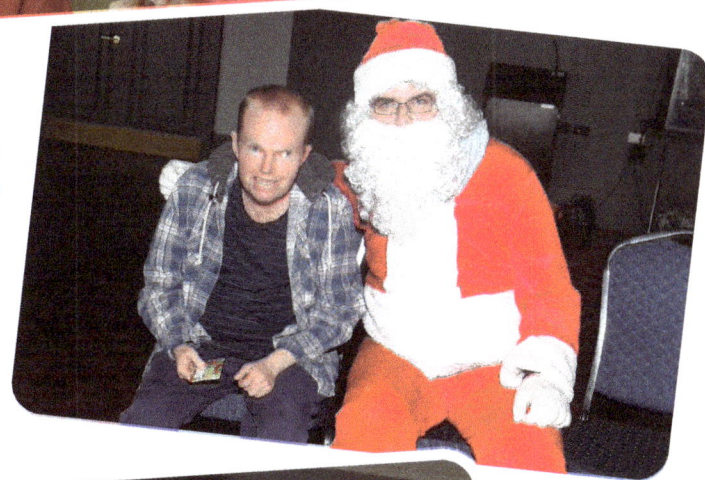

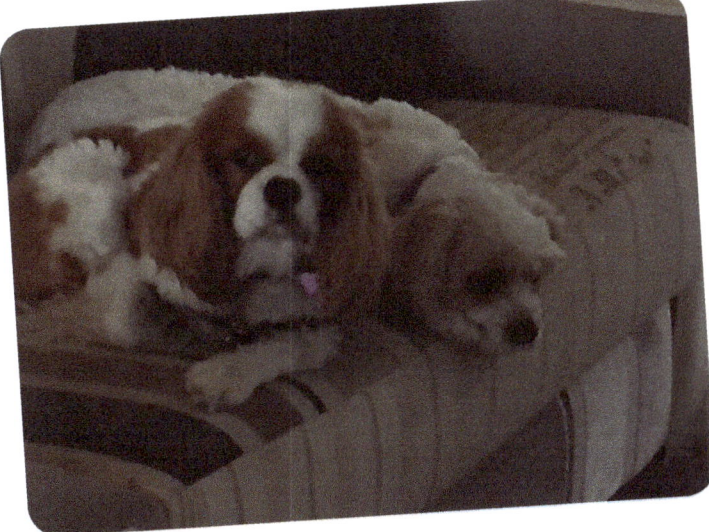

Penny and Bella – the woof whispers 2021

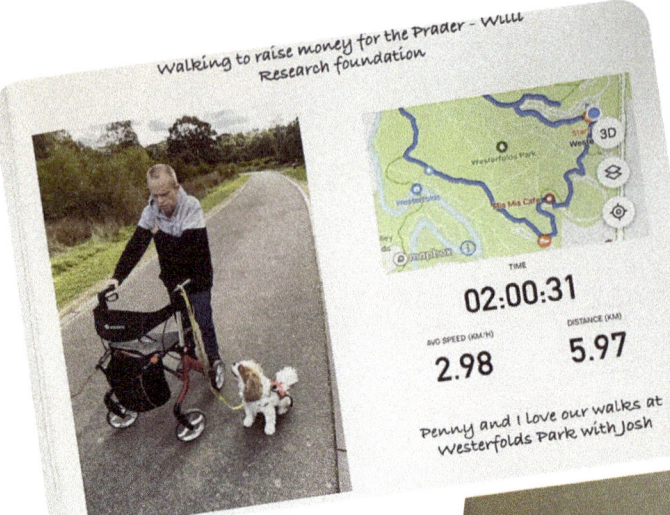

James and Penny walking to raise money for Prader-Will Research Foundation Australia 2023

Bella the woof whisperer with Nanna 2024

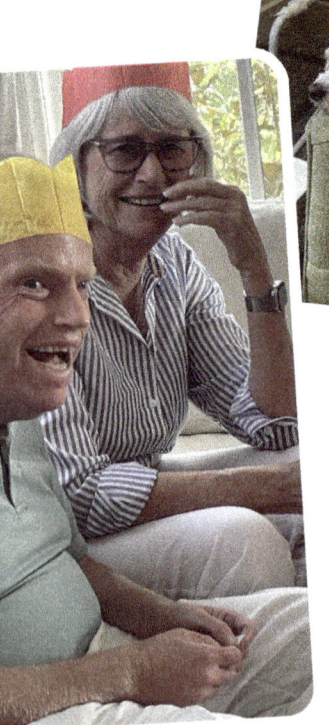

Liz and James Christmas 2024

At the Crossroads

Bearing the burden of caregiver decisions

It is a morning in mid-December 2013. I am sitting in a family meeting room of the Acute Psychiatric Unit of a major Melbourne hospital with my sister Sue and a social worker. The social worker says, 'James needs to be discharged because the doctors say there is nothing more they can do for him as an inpatient.'

With a very breathless and shaky voice, I respond with, 'he doesn't have an address to be discharged to, so he needs to stay here until the Department of Health and Human Services find him suitable supported accommodation.'

I couldn't have stood my ground without the support of my sister and my rehearsed dialogue. Aged 32, James had been admitted via the emergency department to an acute psychiatric unit for the fourth time after a year of unrelenting psychosis despite many antipsychotic medication changes.

> *This is my command – be strong and courageous.*
> *For the Lord your God is with you wherever you go.*
> **Joshua 1:9**

Since arriving in Melbourne three years previously, James had been on a waiting list with the Victorian Department of Health and Human Services (DHHS) for disability supported accommodation. I was repeatedly told that there were no vacancies and that the best they could offer was three hours per week of carer respite funding and two weeks per year of residential respite care.

After talking with other parents who had been in the same situation, I got the strong sense that if a person with a disability had a parent who was upright, with a pulse and breathing, there was little chance of them securing supported accommodation unless there was a crisis such as parent death or disablement.

I was working full-time in a senior academic role at the University of Melbourne and getting help with caring for James between 3pm and 6pm one afternoon from a friend, Ian, at church, from my sister when she could, and from a paid carer another afternoon. Although my academic role allowed for some flexibility in onsite working hours, there were faculty meetings that often ran later than their scheduled finishing time and other unexpected leadership activities that required me to stay at work for extended hours.

James could not cope with any uncertainty about the time I would arrive home so, as the afternoons progressed at work, I became more and more stressed about placing the burden on other people, particularly volunteers and family.

As James' mental health deteriorated, he would often wake several times during the night in a very disturbed state and become physically aggressive. At his worst, he was experiencing auditory hallucinations commanding him to stab me so I had to be vigilant all the time and make sure sharp objects were out of reach at night time.

Life like this became intolerable, with no relief in sight.

After a particularly disturbing night of James trashing his room and trying to break through a top storey window of the house because he was being tormented by auditory hallucinations, I called his psychiatrist who then contacted the Crisis Assessment and Treatment Team. As a result, James endured – and I had to witness – yet another traumatic extraction from home by paramedics and police escorts, a lengthy wait in the emergency department and involuntary admission to the Acute Psychiatric Unit where medications were changed yet again.

Over a three-to-four-week period, James was seen by a few different consultant psychiatrists and several psychiatric registrars who had nothing more to offer except sedating him when he had meltdowns. Numerous antipsychotics had been tried with minimal effect.

During this time, I had been talking with family members, other parents of adults with dual disability and counsellors about how I could continue coping while waiting – possibly for years – for additional government support. The response was the same from everyone, 'refuse to take him home.'

Far from bringing relief, the thought of relinquishing him to government-run care filled me with horror. I am sure that anyone reading this, who has considered putting a spouse in a nursing home or a child of any age into out-of-home care, will recall the awful gut-wrenching reaction despite knowing they can't cope anymore.

Repeated phone calls to DHHS met a consistent response, 'no vacancies in disability supported accommodation; take him home and we'll see if we can find some extra hours of respite.'

Each time a doctor mentioned discharging James, I said I couldn't take him home without guaranteed additional weekly support. Hence, the intervention of the social worker.

Despite the staff in the psychiatric unit observing and recording that James was incapable of performing activities of daily life independently or managing his own medications, the first suggestion from the social worker was to place him in an SRS (supported residential service for patients with mental illness). At that time, residents of an SRS were expected to live independently with a weekly visit from a psychiatric nurse – impossible for James or any other person with Prader-Willi Syndrome!

As Christmas approached, the hospital kept applying pressure on me to take James home. I was not going to give in. Finally, the social worker organised a meeting at the hospital between me and two representatives from DHHS disability supported accommodation. At that meeting, the DHHS reps invited me to view a house not far from where I lived.

My sister Sue and I met them at the address given and it quickly became obvious that the house was vacant and near derelict. There were holes in internal walls, doors swinging on one hinge, leaking taps, broken windows taped up and a putrid smell of rodents. We were told that the house had been unoccupied for months and was being decommissioned by DHHS. They also said it would take a few days to find staff to provide 24-hour care. I was given 48 hours to make a decision.

At that point I was ready to give in and take James home; it broke my heart to think of him living in a place like that. However, Sue suggested that if I refused this place, it might give DHHS the opportunity to label me a difficult or 'picky' mother and move James further down the waiting list. I told DHHS we would take the house and that we would get our church friends to come in and renovate it before moving James.

Amazingly, just 24 hours later, DHHS said there was a vacancy in another house with four other residents just a few suburbs from my home! The contrast between the two houses was huge – this one had been purposefully built for five residents from Kew Cottages after the change in government policy to de-institutionalise people with disability and place them in residential houses. It was spacious, well-appointed, and nicely furnished and decorated. James was transferred from hospital on the 23rd of December. It was only then that I learnt that one of the five original residents of this house had died four months previously, and his room had been vacant ever since!

Had I not made those heartbreaking decisions, first to refuse to take James home from hospital and second to call the bluff of DHHS and accept the derelict house, we could have ended up in the untenable situation of me providing 24-hour care for James with minimal government support for the next six and a half years until the NDIS rolled out in Victoria. Sadly, that was the reality for many families – waiting list after waiting list to get the help they needed.

This is just one of my 'crossroads' experiences, probably the hardest burden to bear, but there have been, and will continue to be, many more.

The decisions don't get easier, but I have become more assertive in standing my ground for James' sake, and my family and faith community have stood beside me.

Negotiating the NDIS

Traversing the everchanging landscape

It is the afternoon of 7 December 2016, and I am sitting at a table in the backyard of James' house with a National Disability Insurance Agency planner. She has a laptop with a preloaded planning document to complete about James' goals and disability-related needs. She tells me she is very new at this, having come from an investment banking background. She admits she has never heard of Prader-Willi Syndrome. A few questions into the process, it becomes obvious that there are set responses to choose from her questions and no capacity to provide explanatory variations. Her advice was to 'just choose the response that describes his worst day, not the best, and not the average.'

Used to taking comprehensive histories from patients to assess their health-related needs, I thought this was a very strange way to go about assessing disability-related needs.

Speak up for people who cannot speak for themselves.
Protect the rights of all who are helpless.
Proverbs 31:8

I had been attending information sessions throughout the year about the rollout of the National Disability Insurance Scheme (NDIS) in Victoria. Some of these sessions were run by National Disability Insurance Agency (NDIA) representatives, and others by Department of Health and Human Services (DHHS) accommodation support personnel. Because James had already been assessed by the Victorian DHHS as fitting the criteria for 'disabled', I knew that he would automatically qualify for the NDIS and continue to be funded for accommodation support, but any other funded supports were to be determined. For example, the day program that James had been attending since 2011 had been receiving block funding from DHHS, but once the NDIS rolled out across Victoria, each participant would need to be assessed and individually funded according to their support needs.

As we progressed through the assessment, I began to realise how important the planner's advice was – this was a black and white process with no shades of grey. Responding that James was sometimes independent or only required occasional prompting to undertake each activity of daily living would not result in sufficient funding for an appropriate level of support during protracted periods of time when his disabilities were unstable and he was unable to function.

These periods were unpredictable in onset and duration.

Having attended the information sessions and read as much as was available on the NDIS website, I also understood the importance of defining acceptable, precise and measurable goals that James would like to achieve with NDIS funded support. This was a practice I was very familiar with from my nursing experience. Governments require measurable outcome data to determine future funding. Additionally, any request for a funded support or service had to be assessed as 'reasonable and necessary' to meet specific disability-related needs – that is, likely to be effective in meeting the participant's goals and not able to be provided or funded by other community or government agencies.

This was a lot to comprehend. I was struggling to understand all the nuances of the scheme and worried that I might miss or underestimate some aspect of James' needs – and I was a well-educated, articulate person with English as my first language! My heart was crying out for families who were unable to access or understand the available information and did not have someone advocating for them.

How would they fare?

Would the scheme and its processes be just and equitable for these families?

In the first few years of the transition from DHHS to NDIS, planning meetings for the subsequent funding period were held face-to-face in a local NDIS office. This enabled James and me, as well as other people who were knowledgeable about his support needs, to attend the meetings with medical and allied health reports and any other data deemed necessary to provide evidence of disability-related support needs.

I experienced these meetings as collaborative and transparent – the planner could ask for further evidence if required and could provide interpretations of any new NDIS policies and procedures, while James and his advocates could seek clarification of any ambiguities or supports not previously known about.

At that time, the only uncertainty was in the response to requests to partly fund the training of an assistance dog. Different planners had diverse interpretations of 'reasonable and necessary'. I wanted to know this because James had started working with the Centre for Service and Therapy Dogs Australia with the goal of having his own assistance dog in the future. He received a small amount of funding in the first plan only, and not the rest. I had heard that the Administrative Appeals Tribunal was dealing with several applications to review overturned requests to fund psychosocial assistance dogs and that the process was onerous and stressful for applicants. I decided not to go down that route.

Sometimes you just have to choose your battles and forego the possible benefit because of the known angst it will cause.

The next hurdle to face was collecting and analysing sufficient credible data to submit as evidence of the need to fund 1:1 support at James' day program. Prior to the NDIS rollout, centre-based day programs received block funding to run its programs and the centre managed this funding to support participants according to their need. That is, some participants could be well supported in a group of four or more with one support worker, while other participants were better supported in a 1:3, 1:2 or 1:1 ratio of staff to participant/s.

In the early years of James' attendance at Araluen Centre, he coped well in a group setting, only occasionally needing more individualised support when emotionally dysregulated. However, as his mental health deteriorated, incident reports of verbal and / or physical aggression increased in frequency. Araluen could clearly demonstrate from their recorded incidents and other daily reports that, when he was in a large group activity, he often became agitated and difficult to manage but when the staff to participant ratio was reduced (particularly if down to 1:1) he was calm, cooperative and fully engaged with his peers.

Was that sufficient data for the NDIA to fund 1:1 day program supports?

No!

For the next two years, significant amounts of NDIS funding were provided for behaviour assessments, interventions and reports by a psychologist in the NDIA's endeavour to establish that James' Prader-Willi Syndrome and mental health behaviours could be modified such that he wouldn't require 1:1 support.

Did that provide the evidence to support NDIA preference to fund at group level and not 1:1?

No; the findings were to the contrary.

The psychologist's reports endorsed Araluen's analyses and conclusions. James did best, other participants were more settled and the staff reported decreased stress levels when he received 1:1 support. With that evidence, the next NDIA planner finally recommended funding for 1:1 support at Araluen and it was granted in his subsequent annual plan.

So, we had two years of James being inadequately supported at group level, day program staff having to manage James' meltdowns while trying to support three or more other participants, and a lot of money spent on assessments and reports to provide data that confirmed evidence previously submitted by Araluen and well described in internationally accepted best practice guidelines for people with Prader-Willi Syndrome.

With NDIS participant numbers increasing each year, the NDIA encouraged participants and their nominees to change from face-to-face to telephone planning meetings. Initially, this was not a problem, because prior notice of date and time was given by the Agency which allowed for the gathering and submission of relevant and required documents to be discussed and clarified during the telephone meeting.

However, that changed. Uncertainty and unpredictability started to creep in. The end date of a funded plan was fast approaching with no notification from the NDIA about the next planning review. Out of the blue, I received a phone call from a NDIA planner announcing a decision to 'roll-over' James' current plan for another year. Two months later, another phone call from a different planner, saying 'sorry, we made a mistake. We can't just roll over plans of participants living in Supported Disability Accommodation. We need to do another review.'

Was that a simple process?

No!

All the service providers had to provide new progress reports and write new service agreements, having only just issued them two months previously. More time wasted and money needlessly expended.

During the Covid-19 lockdowns, funding to providers of supported independent living was based on the assumption that residents would need to stay in their supported disability accommodation homes most days because centre-based day programs had to shut and other community-based activities were suspended. This resulted in the majority of funding being apportioned to supported independent living providers and very little to providers of community-based programs. That was not a problem then, and for the next few years, because funding across supported independent living and other community access activities could be flexibly expended to suit needs and to meet goals as the Covid restrictions eased.

Following the extensive review of the NDIS over the period 2022-2023, changes were made to try and close loopholes in the system that allowed some providers and / or participants to fraudulently claim expenses for services not provided. One such change, brought in towards the end of 2024, was in relation to funding provided for supported independent living – now funded under the category of Home & Living. That support item then became a 'Stated Support', and the funding allocated to that stated support could only be used for that specific support item.

Realising straight away that this change would substantially affect the way James' funding could be spent, I submitted an application for a review of his current plan issued in August 2024 for a 12-month period. It erroneously provided funding in excess of need for Home & Living (the amount was originally calculated during the Covid-19 shutdown period) and a deficit in funding for community access activities – day program, community participation and holiday support. There was no longer any allowance under the new rules to flexibly transfer the excess funds to the category of deficit. I thought to myself, 'should be easy to fix this error… I just need to send the NDIA evidence, in the form of service agreements, invoices and payments to demonstrate exactly how funds had been expended over the past years and the reviewer will see that I am not asking for more funds to enable James to continue his weekly community access activities, just to transfer the excess from Home & Living.'

Poor, deluded me!

The request for review of funding was denied. So, then I had to submit an application for a 'Review of a Reviewable Decision'.

Denied again.

I was not going to give up. This was illogical.

Next attempt to free up the excess funding was to submit a 'Change of Circumstance' form. Four months later, after numerous phone calls, emails and re-submission of reports purportedly lost in the NDIS system, a new plan was issued with a small proportion of the excess funding reallocated to where it was actually needed.

The final report of the NDIS review *Working Together to Deliver the NDIS* (2023 pg 26) noted that, at best, people described the planning process as confusing and frustrating and, at worst, it was described as traumatic. The report also acknowledged that inconsistent and unclear decisions are making participants feel mistrusted, disempowered and angry.

My recent experience indicates that not much has changed. My professional and academic experience has enabled me to find, read and to try and make sense of the constantly changing rules and regulations of the NDIS – but I am flummoxed.

As Rick Norton commented in his Saturday Paper piece about the NDIS, 'no amount of executive function – itself impaired by elevated stress levels – can overcome the peculiar irrationality of the most rational of organisational systems: the government bureaucracy.' (published 1st March, 2025)

Despite the constant stress of negotiating the ever-changing landscape of the NDIS, I am grateful for its existence and the opportunities it provides for James to be supported and meaningfully engaged in his community.

I am also immensely thankful to all the people who have advocated for, and defended, the rights and choices of people with disabilities to live a more ordinary life.

The Woof Whisperers

Encountering the power of canine companionship

It is 10 November 2017, and I am at James' house with Sharon, a dog trainer from the Centre for Service and Therapy Dogs Australia; Penny, a very cute little Cavalier King Charles dog; and James. Sharon has said to James several times, 'Penny is now your dog'.

With each repeated announcement from Sharon, James' responses change from wide eyed, open mouthed, stunned silence through exclamations of 'not really' with a little grin, to a look of rapturous joy and murmurs of 'she's mine, she's mine!'

Dear little Penny just sat on his lap with her nose nuzzled into his chest. Those precious moments are etched in my memory to recall every time I am overwhelmed with other unpleasant images and sounds of James in distress.

Two are better off than one, because together they can work more effectively.
If one of them falls down, the other can help him up.
But if someone is alone and falls, it's just too bad, because there
is no one to help him.
If it is cold, two can sleep together and stay warm,
but how can you keep warm by yourself?
Ecclesiastes 4:9-12

Twenty months prior to this event, I had met with the founder of the Centre for Service and Therapy Dogs Australia (CSTDA), Yariv, to discuss the possibility of James joining their program, 'Dogs for Life'.

My interest was sparked after watching a news broadcast about their work in schools providing dog therapy to children with autism and intellectual disability. Teachers and parents of the children unanimously agreed that they had witnessed a reduction in stress and anxiety in the children, and that aspects of socialisation with each other had improved. Further reading about this program identified its benefits for people with treatment-resistant mental health conditions, particularly post-traumatic stress.

Because James suffered from all these conditions, I thought it was worth investigating.

James had always loved dogs and we had one, Molly, in Queensland before we moved to Melbourne. We couldn't bring Molly with us because she was a great escaper and was becoming less and less able to be left alone when we were out at work and programs. Our good friend Robert from church offered to take Molly so that James was able to receive regular photos and updates about how she was faring.

When we first moved to Melbourne and were initially living with my sister and her husband, James was pleased to have the company of their dog, Moose – a big, black, placid labrador. Together, they would amble around the quiet backroads of Eltham where there was little danger from traffic and a familiar route to follow.

Moving from there to our house 18 months later left James yearning for canine companionship.

When James moved into supported accommodation in 2013, I asked if he could have a pet dog and was very quickly told that he couldn't because other residents were afraid of them. Having explained this dilemma to Yariv, he said their dog trainers were experienced in desensitising fearful people and could work with the other residents if the house staff were agreeable. After a few meetings with Yariv, they agreed to give it a trial.

Yariv outlined Dogs for Life as an animal assisted empowerment program that entailed the participant working with an experienced trainer and service dog to learn the fundamentals of looking after a dog, walking safely in the community and commands to give to the dog. Once these things had been achieved, the trainer and Yariv would start the process of purchasing and training a dog to suit the participant.

We decided to tell James that he was going to start having dog therapy once a week, with no mention of the possibility of him eventually having his own assistance dog, just in case it didn't work out for him or the other residents could not overcome their fears.

Initially, Sharon came to James' house with her dog Perfy to socialise with all the residents. Perfy, as her names suggests, was the perfect choice of dog for this role as she was quiet, calm and very responsive to the residents' reactions – she came close for a pat if invited, but kept her distance if she detected fear. Gradually, they all got used to Perfy's visits and the fear dissipated once they trusted that she was not going to harm them.

The next stage was walking around the local community, with James leading Perfy and Sharon alongside giving instructions and support. As James became confident in his control of Perfy, they ventured into more public areas like parks, coffee shops and shopping centers.

James really enjoyed his 'dog therapy'.

After about eight months, Sharon started bringing other dogs for James to work with. Unbeknownst to him, she was trialing different breeds, sizes and temperaments to assess how well each dog and James bonded. James thought he was helping Sharon train new dogs for Dogs for Life. One day, Sharon arrived with Penny, who was only six months old and being fostered by one of their workers.

I knew that Penny was Sharon's choice for James, but we kept it to ourselves while the intensive training program continued.

As the months rolled by, we could see the bond between James and Penny strengthening. The other house residents appeared to be accepting of Penny coming and going from the house, and the house staff seemed to be agreeable to the guidelines drawn up by Dogs for Life for Penny to be integrated into the house.

The date was set, 10th November, to tell James that after all his dog therapy and training, he was ready to have his own assistance dog.

At the end of 2016, I retired and within a month had purchased my own little fur baby, Bella – a cavoodle. Accompanying Sharon and James on their dog training sessions had given me a lot of insight about dog behaviour and methods of training, so I was well prepared for the delights of puppyhood. Bella and Penny had been born within weeks of each other and I was looking forward to seeing how well they would bond.

The big day arrived. Sharon, James, Penny and I returned to James' house after a training session and, instead of Sharon leaving with Penny as usual, she placed Penny in James' lap and said, 'Penny is now your dog; she can stay here with you and sleep on your bed.'

Needless to say, after the initial jubilation, reality set in dealing with the practicalities of having multiple support workers in the house, each with their own experiences, beliefs and attitudes about handling a dog. However, despite a few hiccups, assimilation of Penny into the house progressed quite well.

Training with Sharon continued for another 18 months with slow, but positive, progress towards James' program goals, which were to:

- develop responsibility, empathy, caring and focus through daily care of Penny
- reduce loneliness and isolation
- provide a companion and purpose for life
- provide a conduit for conversation with people in his community using Penny as a talking point

- enhance capacity to build relationships by translating his bond with Penny onto others
- draw positive attention from others
- provide varied sensory input from Penny as a calming and distracting activity during anxiety and stress
- improve physical fitness, coordination and balance through walking with Penny
- promote settled sleep by the companionship and sensory input of Penny.

Even though Penny always wore her yellow 'Service Dog in Training' coat when out with James, she attracted attention from adults and children alike, probably because she is small and very adorable. Everyone wanted to pat her, and it was good to hear James have the confidence to explain that she couldn't be patted while she was training. He looked every bit the chuffed, proud dog handler.

The next big hurdle was for Penny to pass her Public Access Test so she could be certified as a Service / Assistance dog. She did, and she graduated from wearing her yellow training coat to her red certified service dog coat. What an achievement that was for both Penny and James, not to mention Sharon who did all the hard preparatory work! Penny was now ready to fly – not literally, but permitted to accompany James on a plane for interstate holidays with Wow Tours.

With excited (but nervous) anticipation, James and Penny set out for their holiday on the Gold Coast and Penny's introduction to James' Nanna and Pa at Banora Point. I went with them on the plane and was very relieved to see Penny settle on the floor close to James with not even a stir when the plane took off and landed.

What an intrepid little plane traveler she was!

Well, that was the first trip – returning wasn't quite as uneventful.

At the Gold Coast airport, going through the security check, Penny must have had a bit of the travel jitters because she pooped all the way through. James was non-plussed, Wow Tours support workers were busy with other members of the group so I was left to clean up, much to the amusement of other travelers. Fortunately, the airport security staff were understanding and helpful because I was fearing that we would all be kicked out and not allowed to travel with Penny. Once on the plane, she behaved beautifully and was given lots of pats by the flight attendants.

I was very relieved to arrive back in Melbourne.

The integration of Penny into James' daily life and his home was assisted by comprehensive guidelines from Dogs for Life for the house staff to follow. They included instructions to safeguard Penny if James became verbally and / or physically aggressive because of a mental health breakdown, but also how to re-engage Penny with James to provide comfort to him as he recovered. In addition to Sharon, the dog trainer, a Dogs for Life employed psychologist developed a program to help with his emotional regulation, sensory integration and social engagement.

One of the aims of the Dogs for Life program is for the dog to be perceived not just as an assistance dog, but as a partner to the participant. The dog becomes a 'significant other' in their life. This is sometimes not recognised or accepted by others. An example of this is when house staff have separated Penny from James, because he has become emotionally dysregulated, and he has called out for his 'wife'. This has been reported by staff as an indication of delusional thought processes rather than understanding that this is James' only way of expressing his emotional attachment to Penny.

Being separated from Penny – his significant other – removes a stable, grounding element in his life.

Penny and my dog Bella hit it off right from first meeting, so it was great for James, me and the dogs to go walking together in local parks. Having Bella provided a common interest for James and I as we swapped stories about our dogs and their individual personalities.

I had to keep it a secret from Bella that Penny was allowed into cafes, movie theatres and just about anywhere that James was going, while she had to stay home!

After learning so much from Dogs for Life about the therapeutic psychosocial benefits of dogs, I began to experience it for myself. Bella has become my constant companion, curled up on my lap whenever I am sitting, lying across my feet at night – much better than a hot water bottle – and listening while I prattle on about all sorts of both serious and inane issues. Bella senses when I am not feeling good and snuggles in close, looking at me intently with her big brown eyes.

There is now so much evidence-based information about dogs' abilities to instinctively sense, and respond to, their owners' emotions. Bella has given me unconditional love and provided just the therapy I have needed on many occasions when I have felt like I couldn't bear the burden of James' suffering any more.

As I write this in 2025, I see Bella having this same effect on my 100-year-old mother who lives with dementia. In 2024, my sister Sue and I moved our parents from their nursing home in northern NSW down to one in Melbourne, close to where we both live. At that time, Dad was 102 and Mum was 99. Not long after the move, Dad developed a severe chest infection and died, leaving Mum bereft.

Mum remembers who family members are, but not much more than that. Like other dementia sufferers, she becomes disoriented and agitated. While I am sure she finds our visits to her comforting, she responds best when I take Bella with me. No matter how agitated or tearful she is, once Bella is on her lap, she settles. We can just sit quietly while Mum strokes Bella, remarking how warm and soft she is, often commenting 'Bella loves Nanna.'

Both Penny and Bella have become woof whisperers in times of need.

A dog is someone who knows the song in your heart

and can bark it back to you when you have forgotten the woofs.

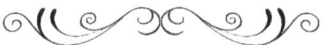

On the Brink

Balancing on a knife edge of physical and mental health relapse

It is around 11pm on 7 October 2018 and I am sitting with a surgical registrar in a large Melbourne hospital. James is being prepared for emergency surgery to deal with another small bowel obstruction – the second in two years. He is critically ill. The registrar is going through the operation consent form with me, carefully explaining the risks and the possibility that he may not survive the surgery. As a registered nurse, I have been privy to such conversations between medical staff and relatives of patients; I know the drill, but this is different – I am now that relative! *Please God, don't let him suffer anymore… take him home if it is your will.*

I have the strength to face all conditions
by the power that Christ gives me.
Philippians 4:13

I don't recall feeling this desperate when James had his first emergency surgery in 2016. That time, he was taken to hospital by ambulance with a grossly distended abdomen, pain, a rapid pulse rate and shallow breathing. This had never occurred before. James had been, physically, quite well up until this time.

After vomiting bowel contents, he was quickly taken for a CT scan of his abdomen which revealed what appeared to be a small bowel obstruction. After an examination by a surgical registrar in the Emergency Department, he was prepared for immediate surgery. Although this was emergency surgery, none of the medical staff appeared to be too concerned. However, they did say he would be going to the Intensive Care Unit (ICU) post operatively because he wouldn't be out of recovery until the early hours of the morning and would need close monitoring for a day or two.

This was James' first hospital admission to anything but an acute psychiatric ward. At that time, I felt way more in control of my fear. I had spent many years working in surgical wards and high dependency units so I knew what to expect in terms of post operative procedures and ward routines. This was familiar territory, unlike that of the acute psychiatric units which felt chaotic and unpredictable.

That 'day or two' in ICU ended up being 10 days because James' bowel was very slow to start functioning again and the intensive care medical staff, with advice from the hospital liaison psychiatrists, decided to keep him sedated until it was medically safe for him to take fluids and food orally.

All people with Prader-Willi Syndrome have a preoccupation with food and a compulsion to eat. This compulsion over-rides everything including abdominal pain and a partial or complete bowel obstruction. Being conscious and not being able to drink or eat would have been intolerable for James.

All people with Prader-Willi Syndrome are also highly anxious, all the time. Any uncertainty about food – when, what, how – increases their stress and results in challenging behaviours for carers (in this case, nurses) to manage.

After transfer from the ICU to the surgical ward and a successful transition from intravenous to oral diet, James was discharged home. The findings from this surgery were that his small bowel was not mechanically obstructed but had just stopped functioning – medically termed a paralytic ileus – principally because of the adverse effects of a particular antipsychotic medication he was taking, and exacerbated by the low muscle tone that is characteristic of Prader-Willi Syndrome.

At that time, there was no suggestion from any of the medical personnel that this was anything but a 'once-off' occurrence, but it was recommended by the surgeons that the psychiatrists find an alternative antipsychotic with less adverse effects on his bowel.

Prior to the next surgery in 2018, James was once again taken to the Emergency Department by ambulance with abdominal pain and distention. An abdominal CT scan looked much like the previous one in 2016, but this time he was admitted to a surgical ward for observation in the hope that the obstruction might resolve by remaining nil by mouth and having a nasogastric tube inserted to decompress his bowel. However, multiple attempts to insert the nasogastric tube resulted in James vomiting and aspirating stomach and bowel contents into his lungs.

Over the next 24 hours, James' vital signs deteriorated to the point of nursing staff making several 'Code Blue' calls. These calls summon the Medical Emergency Team (MET) for rapid assessment and / or resuscitation measures if required. After the third call, it was determined by the surgical team that he needed urgent surgery.

I had been with James through each of the MET calls and had been included in all the discussions between medical staff. I knew he was critically unwell and could see how distressed he was. Even though he is hearing impaired and intellectually disabled, I was fairly sure that he understood what was happening to him, particularly after he asked me, 'am I going to die?'

Trying to reassure him that he was being well cared for while trying to listen to all the medical and nursing 'chatter' was very stressful. I felt shaky and light-headed – probably not helped by lack of food and drink while all the drama was happening.

Thankfully, I had my ever calm and ever supportive sister Sue with me, who ministered to my stress both practically and spiritually. She had alerted our church prayer group and I knew they would all be praying for James and me to be at peace, as well as for the surgical and anaesthetic team to be vigilant and considered in their care of James.

Just like the first time in 2016, James survived the surgery and was transferred to the ICU. He remained there for a week, intubated and ventilated, until his bowel started functioning again and the pneumonia that he had developed from aspirating stomach contents pre-operatively started to resolve. During this time, I was happy to just visit him once a day for a short time, confident that he was receiving around-the-clock 1:1 care and relieved to know that he was unaware of his surroundings or condition.

Being transferred from ICU to the ward was a very traumatic time for both James and me. James remembered the previous hospitalisation and surgery for bowel obstruction and was aware that consumption of food would be very restricted. The anxious questions started the minute he entered the ward: 'Will I just get the brown soup?' 'How long 'til I can have yoghurt?' 'Will the lady with the tea trolley know not to give me biscuits?' 'I'll die without food, won't I?' 'When can I go home?'

Initially, James was placed in a four-bed ward close to the nurses' station. The sickest patients were put there so they could be easily observed by the nurses. I understood this, but I also knew it would create distress for James watching as other patients were brought food from the food trolley and he was not.

I had to stay with him.

As the days rolled on, and the outbursts from James intensified, he was eventually moved to a single room and occasionally the hospital supplied a mental health nurse to stay with him while I got a few hours' break.

Many discussions were held between the surgical team and the psychiatric liaison team – the former wanted him off the antipsychotic medication known to significantly decrease gut motility, and the latter reiterated that many other antipsychotics had been tried in the past with little beneficial effect. The offending antipsychotic, commenced three years previously, had given James relief from psychosis and reduced his anxiety. Since the last admission, attempts had been made to wean James off this medication, but each time he had a psychotic relapse.

So, damned if you do and, likely, damned if you don't!

Finally, James was well enough for discharge home, still on the same antipsychotic with a slightly reduced dose, a modified fiber diet and increased bowel medications. The goal was to try and gradually swap over to other antipsychotics with less effects on gut motility.

Two years later, after several unsuccessful trials of changing antipsychotics and three further admissions for functional bowel obstructions, the decision was made to permanently cease the antipsychotic that had initiated the paralytic ileus problem. Its adverse effects were life-threatening but, without it, James was left with chronic relapsing psychosis and the psychiatrists were left with trying to find a cocktail of other antipsychotics and anxiolytics to give him some relief without exacerbating his bowel issues.

As I write this in 2025, James has been admitted to hospital via the emergency department for functional bowel obstructions another seven times. All these admissions were managed medically, not surgically, with nasogastric tube insertion, initial fasting and then the process of gradually introducing fluids before recommencing solid food. The usual trauma of disrupted food security accompanied every admission.

Some of these admissions were during the Covid lockdowns, so I had to go through the process of getting special permission to be with James in the hospital. If I needed to stay with him past 9pm, I was afraid all the way home of being stopped by the police for being out during curfew. No other family member was allowed into the hospital, and the hospital was short staffed so it was up to me to provide the consistent emotional support he required. I knew that if I wasn't present, meltdowns would occur and physical restraint would be applied – traumatic for both James and staff.

Twelve months ago, James' gastroenterologist recommended that second daily enemas be given to him to mitigate his very poor bowel function. This was considered to be less of a risk to him than surgically inserting a venting tube into his stomach or small bowel. A very challenging characteristic of Prader-Willi Syndrome is chronic skin picking, so there was a concern that James might pick around the tube insertion site if the skin was irritated. Worse still, he could pull the tube out during a meltdown and end up with peritonitis.

Meanwhile, the unrelenting anxiety and psychotic relapses are managed to the best of everyone's abilities with strategies developed by James' behaviour support practitioner and implemented by all the members of his support team. Increasing his antipsychotic medication is a last resort because of its potential to further decrease his already slow gut motility. Everyone has a vested interest in keeping his gut happy.

The balancing act goes on, and on, and on…

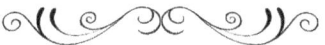

Taking a Stance

Advocating amidst the shadows of recrimination

It is 5 May 2023 and I am sitting in the consulting room of a psychiatrist who is reviewing James' severe deterioration in mental health. Also in the room is James, his nurse case manager and his behaviour support practitioner. James is shaking and crying uncontrollably, repeating over and over, 'she's my dog, she's my dog… why can't I have my dog back?'

The psychiatrist exclaims, 'this is so cruel. Who do I need to write to about this?'

Arms around James, I lead him out of the room to face another day of heartache. Nothing could console him.

*If you listen to me, you will know what is right, just and fair.
You will know what you should do.*
Proverbs 2:9

What had led to this devastating scenario?

Just over two months previously, I received a phone call from staff at James' house informing me that there had been an unexpected visit from two RSPCA inspectors. They had come in response to an anonymous caller who claimed that James' dog Penny was being mistreated by him.

The house staff denied any knowledge of who the caller was and said they had not witnessed or reported any incidents of cruelty towards Penny. Nevertheless, the RSPCA inspectors told the house staff that they would be individually and corporately prosecuted if the complaint was substantiated.

Since I didn't know if the anonymous caller to the RSPCA would make any further complaints, I decided it would be safer for Penny to be go to a Dogs for Life training and boarding facility while we tried to get to the bottom of the issue. Thinking this would be just for a short period of time, I told James that Penny needed to go to 'boot camp' for some re-training.

Initially, he accepted this explanation for her absence and, over the next two weeks, he visited her a few times which provided an opportunity for the trainer to make an assessment of their bonding and of Penny's reactions to James. The trainer's written assessment stated that he had witnessed signs of a strong bond between them and that Penny did not exhibit any anxiety or resistance to James.

I contacted one of the RSPCA inspectors who had visited the house to ask for the details of the complaint. The only detail she would tell me was that the complainant said that James had tried to strangle Penny and Penny was yelping. The inspector would not say if this person had witnessed the event or been told about it by someone else.

A month after Penny's removal from the house, I met with the house supervisor and two managers of the organisation that provided James' supports in the house. Although they had no evidence of any cruelty to Penny and assumed that the complainant was a casual worker from an agency, their focus was on the risk of prosecution to their organisation rather than on the detriment to James' mental wellbeing from being separated from Penny. They said Penny could not return until they had completed a risk assessment.

All of my phone calls and emails to the regional general manager of the organisation requesting information about the risk assessment and Penny's return to the house fell on deaf ears; no response at all. The other two managers who had attended the previous meeting also did not respond to any of my attempted communications. For me, it was like being confronted with a 'code of silence'.

In desperation, I emailed the regional general manager again just before Easter:

> *'Good morning XXXX,*
>
> *Following a conversation with a delegate of the Office of the Public Advocate, I would like to put the following statements and request to you.*
>
> *[Supported Independent Living provider] knowingly and willingly took over care of residents in houses from DHHS with an assurance that those residents would continue to receive all of their current supports. My son, James, had a number of specific health plans and supports in place – including a psychosocial support dog, Penny – because of complex disability and mental health conditions, partly funded by James' NDIS plan.*
>
> *My son had a mental health plan, a behaviour support plan and an animal assisted empowerment program, prescribed by a psychiatrist and a psychologist. These plans described specific guidelines and actions that staff were to take to support James' mental health and general wellbeing while safeguarding Penny*

if James' behaviour became heightened and there was any risk posed to her.

Support dog Penny has played an integral role in regulating James' mental health, particularly as multiple trials of medications have been less than effective or have resulted in numerous hospital admissions – including two in ICU – from life-threatening side effects. As a certified service dog, Penny has previously accompanied James on holidays, to medical and allied health appointments and all social events with no adverse outcomes.

Over the past few years, I have had email communications, phone conversations and face to face meetings with [SIL provider] personnel raising concerns about their capability to deliver high intensity supports to James with acknowledgement from them of deficits and their pledges to undertake investigations, reviews and remedial actions. In recent months, I particularly raised concerns about the level of support provided to James to care for Penny.

After two consecutive routine veterinary check-ups for Penny last year, I informed house staff that Penny had been diagnosed with hearing impairment.

On the 24th of February, I was made aware of an anonymous report being made to the RSPCA about Penny's welfare and a subsequent visit by two RSPCA inspectors to his house.

On the 1st of March, on the recommendation of the Director of Training Programs for the Centre for Service and Therapy Dogs of Australia (CSTDA), Penny was taken from James' home to one of his training sites in Oxley Victoria for assessment of her continuing ability to be certified as a service dog and also to protect her against any further complaint from the anonymous source if it appeared to them that nothing was being investigated.

My communication with the RSPCA indicated that they wanted to know if there were any behavioural issues affecting Penny that would preclude her from being certified as a service dog or indicating mistreatment.

A verbal report from the Director of Training at CSTDA indicated that Penny could not be certified because of her hearing impairment, but could continue to be an emotional support dog to James with the same guidelines for support from staff. On receipt of this information, I was informed by the operations manager at [SIL provider] that Penny could not return to the house until a new risk assessment could be undertaken.

At a meeting on the 24th of March with [SIL provider] personnel, I was told that they had been given legislation relating to the RSPCA and informed of their risk of prosecution should any evidence be found of cruelty to Penny. I was also informed that it was the RSPCA's decision to allow Penny back into the house on receipt of a written report from CSTDA. The RSPCA and [SIL provider] were given that report on the 3rd of April which indicated that there was no evidence of cruelty to Penny.

I was informed by email that the RSPCA had given [SIL provider] all of the information requested and that they were no longer involved. However, [SIL provider] personnel have continued to tell me that they were waiting for the RSPCA's decision.

In the current situation, with James being denied one of his most important supports, his human rights are being violated.

James is the victim of a system and service provider unable to deliver the supports they are funded for.

I am requesting your immediate written confirmation that Penny can return to live with James.

Liz.'

The next week, I received the following email:

'Good afternoon Liz,

Following our email exchange from last week, [SIL provider] has reached a decision on whether Penny returns to James' home.

[SIL provider] has considered a range of matters, including reports that were made available to the organisation. Overall, the decision arrived at was based on whether [SIL provider] could guarantee the safety of Penny whilst in our service.

Upon review of all information, it was found that there was insufficient risk mitigation of harm to Penny within the group home; thus, we were unable to guarantee Penny's safety whilst in our service. This has resulted in the exposure of staff and the organisation to animal cruelty prosecution (as advised by the RSPCA).

In light of this, [SIL provider] has decided that Penny cannot return to James' home. The team at Jamess' house will continue to work with yourself, James and all relevant stakeholders to support James to the best of our ability, and to visit Penny as we move forward.

Regards,

XXXX.'

Once again, I requested copies of all the reports and assessments referred to in this email and on which the SIL provider had made this decision.

Again, I received no response, so I lodged a complaint with the NDIS Quality and Safeguards Commission. It was only after this that I was contacted by the SIL provider's Safeguard Manager and then invited to a meeting with the Chief Operating Officer.

It was now four months since Penny's removal from the house.

Just prior to this meeting, Penny had been diagnosed with a congenital neurological condition – Chiari malformation with moderate-severe syringomyelia – which causes pain to her when held / touched around the neck. James had not intentionally caused Penny any harm. Her yelping was the result of James holding her too tightly.

Despite this information and acknowledgement by [SIL provider] that they had-

- violated James' rights of choice and control
- not based their decision on an RSPCA directive or evidence of any cruelty / abuse / neglect by James;
- ignored expert opinion (head trainer from CSTDA and Behaviour Support Practitioner) in favour of one anonymous, unfounded report to the RSPCA based on wrong assumption of cruelty
- denied James the companionship and support of Penny while in their care
- been told that their risk of prosecution was "miniscule".

-it still took another two months until Penny was allowed to return to her home with James.

Was this a happy ending to the six months of torment for James and unceasing advocacy by me?

No!

The SIL provider engaged an external mediator to conduct meetings between me and two of their staff to resolve, what they deemed, 'a breakdown in relationships'. In my mind, this assertion was simplistic and abrogating their accountability for the events of the past six months. However, I agreed to participate in the hope that truths would be revealed which may lead to good outcomes.

Was it a worthwhile experience?

Yes and no!

Over the four months of mediation meetings and communications, I believed that I was listened to and I was able to make sense of why some house-level staff thought that I had 'crossed the line' into a pseudo-management role. I also discovered that we had different ideas about trust. What I heard was that I should simply trust that staff will do a good job and I should step back – whereas for me, trust needs to be based on knowledge and experience; knowing that good systems and processes are in place and are being followed. I come from a professional background of continuous quality improvement, monitored by national and institutional bodies. Although the NDIS are slowly moving into this space, I acknowledged that this may not be familiar to point-of-care disability support workers.

I also heard that the last six years had been 'hell for staff' with transition from DHHS to [SIL provider], the expectations of the NDIS, and the perceived lack of support from senior managers. There appeared to be a sizable disconnect between the rhetoric of the NDIS, the SIL provider and house-level staff.

It became clear to me that I was the scapegoat in their discontent and, while I could logically make sense of this, it hurt.

A positive outcome was an agreement that I would be accepted as an equal member of James' care team along with my knowledge of Prader-Willi Syndrome and James' health conditions.

Overall, the impact on James of having Penny removed from him without his consent or justifiable reason was unrelenting grief from the loss of his companion, loss of trust in house staff, fear of what else might happen to him or be taken away from him, decreased mental health stability and a sense of disempowerment.

For me, the impact was a disrupted life, sadness in seeing James so grief stricken, unrelenting stress at having to advocate for James in a culture of silence and having to go to extreme measures – a complaint to NDIS Quality & Safeguards Commission – to get justice for him, a loss of trust in [SIL provider] to put the welfare and rights of James before their own self-interest, and fear of what else staff might do to vindicate themselves and / or jeopardise Penny's safe assimilation into the house.

Was I alone in my experience of being an advocate for James?

No!

One of the six commissioners on the *Royal Commission into Violence, Abuse, Neglect and Exploitation of People with Disability* commented, at the annual general meeting of a family support group, that a recurring theme arising from both public and private hearings was from families who had been described as 'annoying, picky, a nuisance, litigious and invading their work space' after they had raised concerns and issues directly with disability service providers.

I live in hope that, one day, advocates will be celebrated in the light of justice rather than shunned in the shadow of recrimination.

Fragile Moments

Creating calm amidst the tempest

I am abruptly awoken by the notification sound of FaceTime coming from my mobile phone next to my bed. My pulse rate quickens and I take a deep breath. I know who it will be looking at me from the screen and I brace myself. I pick up the phone and there is his face contorted into a look of terror – just like Edvard Munch's painting *The Scream*. No sound comes from James' mouth.

Another day of torment for him and worry for me.

Peter got out of the boat and started walking on the water to Jesus.
But when he noticed the strong wind, he was afraid
and started to sink down in the water,
'Save me, Lord!' he cried.
Matthew 14:29-30

As James' mental and physical health declined, his fragile moments have increased in frequency and intensity. The trauma of being unwillingly separated from his companion dog Penny for six months contributed significantly to this decline and, although he experienced some relief with her return, he continues to be plagued with paranoid delusions and anxiety-driven intrusive thoughts.

The voiceless scream has become characteristic of James' torment, often accompanied by hands up in the air in front of him in a stance of fending off the 'voices' (auditory hallucinations) he hears.

Over many years, James has become convinced that the day program he was attending also ran a 'disability prison'. In reality, they have a residential home on their site, housing a small group of people with disabilities who also attend the day program. James believes, because his 'voices' keep telling him so, that he will be put in this 'prison' if certain events happen. The list of events is endless – not being picked up from the day program on time, casual staff not knowing where he lives, rules of the day program or his SIL provider changing, me dying…

What is the driving force behind his fear of imprisonment?

There is no food in prisons – according to the voices and James' amplified memories of stories he heard when visiting historic prisons. The ultimate nightmare for a person with Prader-Willi Syndrome!

Withdrawing from the day program, multiple reassurances of his safety, antipsychotic and anxiolytic medications, and 1:1 daily support with a variety of activities have failed to stop the fear. So, all the members of his support team, including me, are entrusted with creating calm amidst the tempest of James' life.

How does this happen?

Over the decades of James' life, international and national Prader-Willi Syndrome associations and research foundations together with health professionals have been tireless in their efforts to better understand how a person with PWS thinks and behaves to enable the development and dissemination of guidelines for parents and carers. These give us the basis on which to build specific plans and processes for the person we are supporting.

Although people with PWS share common characteristics, each person is unique in the degree to which those characteristics are expressed, and in the strengths and weaknesses they may have inherited or acquired from their life circumstances. James, in addition to having the usual PWS characteristic of relentless anxiety, has severe mental illness which intensifies this anxiety, frequently cascading into paranoid delusions.

James has a mental health plan and a behaviour support plan developed by his mental health team and behaviour support practitioner, in collaboration with me and other members of his daily support teams. These plans are regularly reviewed, not just to update any changes in James' health and wellbeing, but to ensure consistency between them. Training is also provided to support staff for them to implement the plans.

Managing transitions between activities and support staff, providing predictability and minimising uncertainty are key to creating the calm. So too is responding to James' anxieties and fears in an empathic, respectful and warm tone. Trying to reason with him is not helpful because, like all people with PWS, he has poor executive functioning.

Looks fairly straight forward on paper, doesn't it?

Well, unfortunately, life is not always predictable – support staff get sick, go on holidays, change jobs; traffic hold-ups cause delays in staff getting to where they need to be; casual staff don't have time or sometimes interest to read and understand care plans; and a pandemic can suddenly change everything we take for granted. Additionally, we all have upheavals and disruptions to our own lives, which can sometimes result in depletion of resilience to remain empathic and positive in the face of a meltdown.

Nevertheless, we keep on keeping on.

James responds much better to visuals than verbal explanations so, each month, I produce a calendar of all his planned activities – doctors and allied health appointments, rosters of support staff taking him out for the day, and family or social events. Oassist workers, who have known James for a long time, manage the day's activities according to his frame of mind. When settled – and to keep him grounded – they go for long walks in parks with Penny, visit coffee shops where they are now familiar faces to the staff, go to the movies, join a local community drop-in centre for music and games, or go to a heated pool for hydrotherapy or just to relax. On days when James is very fragile and unable to focus on any outdoor activities, they will go for long drives listening to James' favourite playlist of songs while acknowledging his fears and assuring him of his safety.

The house staff where James lives try to engage him in household activities, play a video game or watch TV with him – James loves watching sport, particularly the AFL and his favourite team, the Brisbane Lions. Many days, James is too disturbed to engage in anything other than relaxing in a warm bath listening to music. Just like in any group of workers, some are proactive, creative problem solvers and compassionate while others just get the tasks done. James is very intuitive to these different workers and reacts accordingly.

James FaceTimes me regularly and often. When he is very disturbed, the voiceless scream confronts me and he is in no state to comprehend anything I might say to provide comfort. Other times, as soon as I answer, he will launch into a repetitive string of anxious words or phrases – known as disorganised speech, such as 'he won't, won't, won't, won't…' or 'they said, they said, they said, they said…'

Sometimes, there appears to be no sense to these words or phrases but, at other times, I decipher them as James repeating what the voices are saying to him. Some days these scenarios are repeated over and over until either I don't answer the FaceTime call or James is distracted by a support worker at his end.

Very rarely these days, we might have a conversation about football scores or plans for our Sunday outings and, even more rarely, I might glimpse a tiny fleeting smile. Those flashes are precious and grabbed onto as a glimmer of hope that James is feeling safe and connected, at least for that moment in time.

Every Sunday, I pick James and Penny up and we go to church together, then come home to my place for lunch, visit his Nanna in the nursing home, sometimes play a board game and take the dogs for a walk. He is calm and settled in church and particularly enjoys the music. Recently, James has started attending a community drop-in program run by a network of Uniting Churches for people with, or recovering from, mental illness. Once a month, they have a worship service in which the participants pray for each other. He really looks forward to this and seems to derive comfort from his attendance.

Penny still accompanies James on all his activities, even though she is no longer a certified service dog. I bought her a new coat with 'Support Dog' written on it and, so far, no-one has barred her entry to public places usually reserved for certified dogs. Even though she has very little hearing and is quite heavily sedated with medication for her neurological condition, she still seems to be tuned-in to James' state of mind, snuggling in close when he needs a calming influence. It is not just her presence that is calming, but also the weight of her body against him – much like the weighted blanket he has on his bed – recommended by the occupational therapist.

Along with immersion in warm water, rides in a moving vehicle, music and Penny's presence, scented oils diffused in his room or applied to his body also provide a buffer to James' heightened emotions.

Fortunately, for both weight control and mental wellbeing, James has always enjoyed walking which is known to stimulate the release of neurotransmitters that play a role in mood regulation as well as to reduce the stress hormone cortisol. Additionally, walking in parklands provides a distraction from negative thoughts and an opportunity to engage in mindfulness activities like listening for the sounds of birds, frogs and crickets. James needs a lot of help from his support workers to be mindful of his surroundings, but it also gives them a great sense of reward when they see positive results.

What about my fragile moments?

Earlier in this book, I related a time when I awoke one morning to the thought 'I can't do this anymore... I'm going to have a nervous breakdown.'

But then quickly replaced that thought with 'not today, too much to do.'

That was when I was working full-time and constantly summonsed away from work to pick James up from school because the teacher couldn't manage his meltdowns. I have now been retired for many years and I no longer have those competing demands on my time and attention.

However, that first thought lingers.

Just like Peter who responded to Jesus' command to have courage but then faltered as he focused on the tempest around him, I too sometimes falter and allow my negative emotions to take hold with a 'woe is me' grip. I fall into the trap of thinking I need to 'fix' whatever problem or delusion James is experiencing, yet I know that I can't.

My calm is created by knowing that I am not doing this alone. James has a good support team around him and I have a sister with an always listening ear and voice of reason. I also have my dog Bella who provides me with the impetus to get out for a walk and enjoy the calming influence of the flora and fauna that surrounds me. I have been inspired to do this more often after reading Indira Naidoo's 2022 book *The Space Between the Stars – On love, loss and the magical power of nature to heal.* She wrote this after the tragic death of her youngest sister and her discovery of how nature that surrounds us – even in an urban landscape – can heal us.

Sometimes, it is the simplest things like warm water, music, motion, fragrances, trees changing to autumn colours, or a wet canine nose that provide the calm amidst the tempest.

Knocking on Empty

Refilling the resilience tank

It is 10 July 2024 and I am standing in a pit with water up to my neck and rising. I am holding an umbrella up above my head to shield me from torrential rain but I am saturated and fear I will drown. I see a short ladder leaning against the wall of the pit. Do I have the strength to get to it? Is it long enough to climb out?

'Help!'

The Lord is my guide; I have everything I need
He leads me to peaceful places and restores my spirit
Even when I face challenges, I will not fear, for you are with me
You provide comfort and support, and my life overflows with blessings
I will dwell in your presence forever.

Psalm 23

Did this really happen?

Yes, but not literally. I had drawn a picture of this scenario for a session that day I was going to have with a psychologist I had been consulting for a few months. She had asked if I could express my feelings in a creative way other than words – very difficult for me, who would much rather think than feel.

I explained to her what the picture revealed. The torrential rain was the continual stressors of James' declining mental health and increased neediness together with the constantly changing managers, support workers and policies of his Supported Independent Living provider and their abrogation of responsibility all through the trauma of James' involuntary separation from his dog Penny.

The umbrella was my shield that was battered and becoming ineffective. The pit characterised a feeling of being trapped in a situation where I was about to drown. I told her that I felt like my resilience tank was knocking on empty and I needed help to refill it.

Yet, I had drawn a ladder!

Way back when James was only seven years old, I purchased a book titled *The Management of Prader-Willi Syndrome* (PWS), edited by Randell Alexander and Louise Greenswag (1988) and was horrified to read in the foreword that 'parents, usually unable to manage diets, food-seeking activities, and bizarre behavior, become distraught and emotionally drained… life becomes hell for all concerned.'

Alexander had written this foreword as a paediatrician who had witnessed many parents of children with PWS come to his office in great distress and total despair, telling him of their feelings of helplessness. At that time, I did not feel like that – James was not too difficult to manage, I had good support around me and I felt in reasonable control.

Little did I know that, 36 years later, I would fit that description!

Since the publication of that book, there have been hundreds of articles written about PWS and many outline the effects of the syndrome on families – diagnosis-related grief, ongoing feelings of loss, compassion fatigue, guilt, isolation, and increased rates of poor physical and mental health. I have experienced most of these impacts but, fortunately, not all at the same time.

For 43 years I had navigated life with James without any professional counselling, so why did I feel the need now?

Perhaps it was because my father had recently died at age 102, and the partially closed gates that had previously allowed the grief and loss related to James to just trickle out had now opened like floodgates. Or maybe it was because I had previously studied and worked hard which provided an alternate focus to just being James' mother, and now I was retired with no professional responsibility or identity. I could go on with 'perhaps', 'maybe', 'possibly' – but, in the end, it was time to reflect on my life and to weigh up all the strengths and supports that had kept me going over the years, while also considering new strategies to keep me going into the future.

The psychologist gently suggested that the ladder in my drawing might be joined to a whole lot of other ladders above, forming a framework of connections and supports. The more I thought about that, I could identify each ladder – family, social networks, support groups, faith community, lived experience, professional experience, access to information, care team of professionals and support workers. They were all still there.

Just like the African proverb 'it takes a village to raise a child,' many studies have identified that it also takes a village – or community of care – to support someone with a disability. Family, social networks, support groups and my faith community had not withdrawn support from me but I had loosened my connections to them through fear of being a burden, or someone who had nothing interesting to talk about because I was so consumed with trying to find a way to improve James' quality of life. I had the misguided notion that I was responsible for James' wellbeing and that I was failing. It was up to me to reach out and grab the hands of those waiting to help me up the ladder.

I tentatively suggested to the psychologist that writing my story might give me a meaningful project to reoccupy my thinking and time. She agreed wholeheartedly and also suggested that it might be a very cathartic experience. Hence, the writing of this book you are reading.

What was of great help to me at this time was reading some other people's stories, particularly those who had life changing experiences. I started with Julia Baird and her two books: *Phosphorescence – On awe, wonder & things that sustain you when the world goes dark* and *Bright Shining – how grace changes everything*. I also read Indira Naidoo's book *The Space Between the Stars – On love, loss and the magical power of nature to heal*.

Both of these women had suffered immensely – from different circumstances – yet they had found ways to not only survive, but to strengthen their resilience. A commonality between them was to seek awe and nature daily wherever they were. They also validated that, while they could not control what had caused their suffering, they could control the way they responded through self-determination and discipline. Reading their stories also highlighted for me the importance of identifying and using my strengths while accepting that, at times, I am vulnerable and need help.

As a Christian, I have accepted God's grace of complete forgiveness of all my wrongdoings but, reading Julia Baird's second book *Bright Shining* exposed me to how unforgiving and resentful I had become towards those I perceived to have done harm to James. I had not extended grace to them. Holding that bitterness was unhealthy and a barricade to moving on, so, before writing about past hurts and injustices I have reflected on the bigger picture – the power dynamics and social inequalities that were possibly influencing the attitudes, beliefs and behaviours of the perpetrators. That has helped me to think about whether they were serving their own interests, or were perhaps victims of systemic power and control. Either way, I needed to repair the past with forgiveness.

Writing this book has helped me to see how and why I have become resilient and what I need to keep doing to refill the tank when it starts to run low. Looking back through the chapters I have written I can pinpoint specific modes of thinking and behaviours that have both helped and hindered, although I may not have had that insight at the time.

Knowledge has always been very important to me and I have been blessed with many opportunities to engage in formal study and also to learn from wise people. Formal study has given me the skills to access, analyse and synthesise information. I feel more in control when I have at least a smattering of knowledge that I can discuss with professionals about issues affecting James' life. For me, knowledge is the precursor to decision-making about what situations I will accept, adapt to, or fight to change. The downside to this is when I become so absorbed in searching for information that may improve James' life that I lose sight of other things that sustain me – like social connections.

Another challenge to deal with in the quest for solutions to James' ongoing and debilitating physical and mental health problems is accepting that currently there is nothing more than has already been tried. It can be easy to spiral down into despair. At these times, I have to cling on to hope.

Resilience is built again by hoping that all the scientists and clinicians who are working diligently to find treatments for people with PWS and those with mental illness will find some answers. Their efforts are being rewarded in small increments of new knowledge and therapies, and I help in small ways by contributing to family and clinician advisory panels.

My hope also rests in my faith that James will be healed, perhaps not in this life, but his eternal life to come. James believes this also.

Completing tertiary studies and holding down responsible positions has required discipline – to plan and organise my time efficiently, to be prepared, to complete tasks and to learn from mistakes. These have been valuable foundations to building resilience in my life generally, but they are not sufficient. I have had to become disciplined in eating and sleeping well in addition to getting out and enjoying what nature has to offer, as well as practicing grace.

Resilience has also grown from embracing and connecting to meaningful relationships. As mentioned earlier in this book, I have been blessed with many people who have traveled with me on this journey with James. I have learnt from their wisdom and been upheld by their care and compassion. Being part of a circle of shared experience, through membership of family support groups, has also provided insights into how others have coped and thrived in difficult circumstances.

Probably the greatest practice (but hardest to sustain) in building resilience is gratitude. I have much to be thankful for – an understanding and committed extended family, a good education, good health, a comfortable lifestyle, loyal friends, a team of compassionate support workers committed to improving James' wellbeing, and a forgiving God. Yet, at times, I wallow in self-pity, dwelling on the things I have lost or missed out on. It takes discipline and practice to be thankful every day, even if it is just for a small thing.

Having counselling was also a learning experience. I discovered how much I had repressed my emotions over the years – starting back in childhood but increasing during adulthood. Stuffing them down somewhere out of mind and sight erroneously gave me a sense of control and belief that I could think my way out of most situations. I am a slow learner when it comes to allowing myself to be vulnerable!

So, did I climb out of the pit?

Yes, with a lot of reflection on my part and help from others.

The resilience tank is in a constant state of refilling, emptying and refilling again, but I guess that's life!

Divine Assurance

Finding strength through adversity

Deuteronomy 31:6

So be strong and courageous! Do not be afraid and do not panic before them. For the Lord your God will personally go ahead of you. He will neither fail you nor abandon you.

Joshua 1:9

This is my command – be strong and courageous! Do not be afraid or discouraged. For the Lord your God is with you wherever you go.

Psalm 46:1

God is our refuge and strength, always ready to help in times of trouble.

Isaiah 43:2

When you go through deep waters, I will be with you. When you go through rivers of difficulty, you will not drown. When you walk through the fire of oppression, you will not be burned up; the flames will not consume you.

Isaiah 40:31

But those who trust in the Lord will find new strength. They will soar high on wings like eagles. They will run and not grow weary. They will walk and not faint.

Jeremiah 29:11

"For I know the plans I have for you," says the Lord. "They are plans for good and not for disaster, to give you a future and a hope."

Habakkuk 3:19

The Sovereign Lord is my strength! He makes me as surefooted as a deer, able to tread upon the heights.

Romans 5:3-4

We can rejoice, too, when we run into problems and trials, for we know that they help us develop endurance. And endurance develops strength of character, and character strengthens our confident hope of salvation.

2 Corinthians 1:4-5

He helps us in all our troubles so that we are able to help others who have all kinds of troubles, using the same help that we ourselves have received from God.

2 Corinthians 12:9

My grace is all you need, for my power is greatest when you are weak.

Philippians 4:13

I can do all things through Christ who gives me strength.

Colossians 1:11

We also pray that you will be strengthened with all his glorious power so you will have all the endurance and patience you need. May you be filled with joy.

2 Timothy 1:7

For God has not given us a spirit of fear and timidity, but of power, love, and self-discipline.

James 1:3

For you know that when your faith is tested, your endurance has a chance to grow.

Adversity is something everyone experiences, and most of us turn to someone or something for comfort and guidance when facing these challenges. Like most people, I turn to family, friends and support groups. As a Christian, I also turn to the Bible and throughout the Old and New Testaments there are numerous verses about trials, tribulations, suffering, hope, strength and power. I have provided just a few.

Do I believe them?

Yes.

Do I always live by them?

No, but I keep coming back to these verses. There is something very comforting and reassuring about these divinely inspired messages. However, there have been many times, when in the midst of a crisis, I have railed against God in anger, frustration and disappointment, asking 'where are you God? Why don't you do something? Why God, why?'

But, at other times I have remained calm, resolute and confident that, not only does God hear and know, but he is right there in the midst of it all with me. Reflecting now on the drawing I did for the psychologist – mentioned in a previous chapter – I can envisage God being with me in the pit, perhaps as a life jacket keeping me afloat.

Adversity often feels like a storm, relentless and overwhelming. Yet, within its tempest, divine assurance stands as a lighthouse, unwavering and bright. For me, God's presence offers an anchor amid suffering, a quiet voice reminding me that hardship is not the end of the journey but a passage toward something greater. It is in these trials that my faith is tested and refined, resilience is strengthened, and hope is rekindled. In despair, I can sometimes feel abandoned, but the Bible tells me that even in the darkest valleys, I am never alone.

Suffering, though painful and wounding, has the power to transform. It has stripped away most of my illusions and distractions, leaving behind a deeper understanding of what truly matters to me. Despair has taught me to appreciate the smallest of joys – a kind word, music, a walk in the park, the sound of a bird chirping, the loving look in my dog's eyes. Through all my bleak times with James, I have learnt to become more compassionate, more tolerant and more aware of the struggles of others. With hindsight, I think that suffering has also produced strength and wisdom.

My wounds have become my unforeseen blessings; without them I may never have found faith or deep compassion for individuals and families impacted by disability or mental illness. I am drawn to the vulnerable and those who often dwell on the fringes of our communities, and I have empathy for people who struggle to find or keep faith when they are in the pit of suffering. Suffering through these wounds has developed resilience and endurance in me. It has also shaped my perceptions of others' worth and my belief in the strength of 'community'.

Have my wounds healed?

I think so but, like all wounds, scars have been left and I am mindful that these scars are vulnerable and could break down if I don't take care of them.

What does 'taking care' look like?

For me, it is keeping physically healthy and fit, valuing and sustaining relationships with family and friends, nourishing my spirit by giving to and receiving from a nurturing faith community and seeking joy in music, outings and nature.

Although fairly rare these days, even a tiny glimmer of a smile from James or a little chuckle brings a feeling of elation, because they are signs that he is not just existing but experiencing an inner calm or peace that has surpassed his intrusive thoughts and anxieties – perhaps just for the moment. It is these moments that remind me that God has not abandoned him either.

Divine assurance does not promise a life without trials, but it does promise that no trial is faced in isolation. The promise of redemption and of renewal reminds me that despair is not permanent. What is broken can be made whole, what is lost can be restored, and through it all, joy and hope can be close companions.

My story of adversity is not an isolated struggle but a thread woven into the tapestry of God's larger story. Throughout scripture and human history, hardship has often been the soil in which growth, redemption, and purpose take root. When I encounter suffering, it's easy to feel as though I am lost or forgotten, but within God's narrative, adversity is often a chapter leading to transformation, revealing his faithfulness and deepening my trust in him.

From Joseph's betrayal and imprisonment, to David's years of exile and Paul's imprisonment, biblical figures faced trials that seemed unfair and overwhelming. Yet, in each case, their suffering was not the end of the story – it became the means through which God shaped them for greater purposes.

These examples remind me that God does not waste our pain; he repurposes it, using it for his glory and our good. When we surrender our pain to him, he weaves it into something beautiful – perhaps not in ways we expect, but in ways that ultimately bring restoration, wisdom, and a deeper connection with him.

I often feel like I am stumbling along this path and have fallen a few times, but I am not going to take a detour.

I have learnt that it is not sufficient to merely survive each crisis episode; it is necessary to learn from what the experience has had to teach. I have been confronted with the reality that, because of the nature of PWS, my son's physical and mental health rest on a very fragile veneer of stability; that life can change in an instant; that there have been and will continue to be times of feeling helpless and hopeless; that I have not only survived many crises in James' life but have grown through them; I have experienced love and support from family, friends and God. I have sometimes questioned where God has gone, but hold on to his promises.

I know that the next time I am confronted with James' mental suffering, a failed treatment or an unjust system, I may initially react negatively and feel despair, frustration, annoyance (and possibly anger), and I will probably rail at God again. After wallowing for a while in self-pity and doubt, I will listen to that quiet inner voice that says 'I am with you; I have not left you.'

I will go back and read the words I have written above to still myself, take a deep breath and acknowledge that my experiences have shaped me into a resilient advocate for James and a contributor – in a small way – to a better understanding of the life of someone with lifelong disability and mental illness and those who care for them.

www.ingramcontent.com/pod-product-compliance
Lightning Source LLC
Chambersburg PA
CBHW061221070526
44584CB00029B/3929